Super Easy

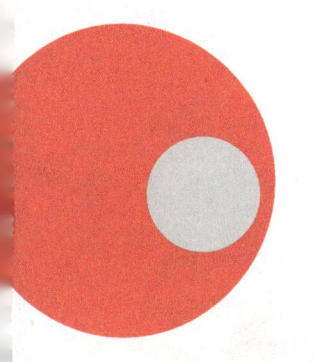

PREDIABETIC COOKBOOK AND MEAL PLANS

Simple Satisfying Meals to Reduce Insulin Resistance, Regain Energy, and Promote Metabolic Balance

Vivian Rose Ellington

COPYRIGHT

All rights reserved. No part of this book may be reproduced, distributed, or transmitted in any form or by any means, including photocopying, recording, or other electronic or mechanical methods, without the prior written permission of the publisher, except in the case of brief quotations used in reviews or other noncommercial uses permitted by copyright law.

DISCLAIMER

The recipes and techniques shared in this book are based on the author's personal experience and culinary expertise. While every effort has been made to ensure the accuracy and reliability of the information provided, the author and publisher make no guarantees regarding the success or outcome of the recipes when followed. The author and publisher disclaim any liability for any damages, losses, or injuries resulting from the use of these recipes. Readers should exercise caution and adjust recipes to suit their individual dietary needs, preferences, and cooking equipment. Always consult a healthcare professional or nutritionist before making significant changes to your diet.

Table of Contents

- Introduction 4-6

- **Chapter 1:** Foods to Avoid 7-10

- **Chapter 2:** Breakfast: A Fresh Start to Your Day 11-19

- **Chapter 3:** Lunch: Keeping Your Energy Stable 20-28

- **Chapter 4:** Dinner: Recipes 29-37

- **Chapter 5:** Vegetarian Recipes (Plant-Based) 38-46

- **Chapter 6:** Appetizers and Salads 47-55

- **Chapter 7:** Soups and Stews 56-64

- **Chapter 8:** Fish and Seafood 65-73

- **Chapter 9:** What to Eat for Prediabetes Management 74-79

- **Bonus:** Your 28-Day Meal Plan 80-85

- Conclusion 86-88

Introduction

WELCOME TO A HEALTHIER YOU

Welcome to Super Easy Prediabetic Cookbook and Meal Plans! First off, I want to congratulate you for taking the first step toward a healthier future. Whether you've just been diagnosed with prediabetes or are looking for ways to manage your blood sugar, you've made a powerful choice. This cookbook is here to guide you through the process of better health with easy-to-follow, nutritious meals that will make you feel your best without overwhelming you with complicated instructions or hard-to-find ingredients.

I know that the idea of managing your health through diet can feel daunting. There's so much information out there, and it's easy to feel like you're not sure where to begin. But I'm here to tell you that it's much simpler than you think. By making small, manageable changes to what you eat, you can feel more energized, reduce your blood sugar, and even work towards reversing your prediabetes all while enjoying delicious, satisfying meals.
This is your journey, and I'm excited to walk alongside you every step of the way.

UNDERSTANDING PREDIABETES: WHAT IT MEANS AND WHY IT MATTERS

Let's start with the basics. Prediabetes is a condition where your blood sugar levels are higher than normal but not high enough to be classified as type 2 diabetes. Essentially, it's a warning sign that your body is starting to have trouble processing sugar efficiently. But here's the good news: just because you're in the prediabetes stage doesn't mean you have to develop diabetes.

With the right lifestyle changes, particularly diet and exercise, prediabetes can often be reversed. The key here is early intervention. By taking action now, you have the power to control your health and prevent the progression to type 2 diabetes.
In this book, we'll show you how to make smart food choices that stabilize your blood sugar levels and support your body's natural processes. It's not about making huge sacrifices; it's about making small, sustainable changes that will have a lasting impact on your health

THE POWER OF DIET: HOW THE RIGHT FOODS CAN HELP MANAGE PREDIABETES

You might be surprised to learn just how much diet plays a role in managing your blood sugar. The foods you choose to eat can either help balance your blood sugar or send it on a rollercoaster ride. But don't worry this doesn't mean you have to give up the foods you love.

The key is balance. By incorporating more whole grains, lean proteins, healthy fats, and fiber-rich vegetables into your meals, you can keep your blood sugar levels steady throughout the day. This book is designed to help you understand what foods work best for your body, and more importantly, how to prepare them in ways that are simple, delicious, and satisfying.

You don't have to become a master chef overnight, but by making small, nutritious choices, you'll start feeling the difference almost immediately. You'll have more energy, better focus, and even experience fewer cravings for those sugary snacks.

HOW TO USE THIS BOOK: YOUR GUIDE TO EASY, BALANCED MEALS

This cookbook is your ultimate guide to managing prediabetes through food. Inside, you'll find easy-to-follow recipes, a comprehensive meal plan, and helpful tips for creating balanced meals that support your health. Here's how to get the most out of this book:

- **Follow the 28-Day Meal Plan:** This meal plan is designed to kickstart your journey. It's a step-by-step guide that takes the guesswork out of meal planning. You'll find a mix of breakfast, lunch, dinner, and snacks to keep you satisfied and energized throughout the day.
- **Use the Recipes:** Every recipe is crafted to be easy, healthy, and full of flavor. You'll find that managing your blood sugar doesn't mean eating bland food. With ingredients you can find at your local grocery store, these meals are designed to work for your lifestyle.
- **Focus on Balanced Meals:** Throughout the book, you'll learn about the importance of balanced meals that combine fiber, protein, and healthy fats. Each recipe is built around this principle, so you don't have to worry about complex calculations just eat, enjoy, and feel great.

Remember, this book isn't about perfection. It's about making better choices every day, and feeling good while doing it.

TIPS FOR SUCCESS: SMALL CHANGES, BIG RESULTS

The journey to better health doesn't happen overnight, but that doesn't mean you can't make big strides with small changes. Here are a few tips to help you succeed:

- **Take it One Meal at a Time:** Don't overwhelm yourself by thinking about everything at once. Focus on each meal and make it the best choice for your health.

- **Plan Ahead:** Meal prepping is one of the easiest ways to stay on track. Prepare your meals in advance, and you'll have healthy options ready to go when you need them.

- **Don't Stress Over Perfection:** It's okay to slip up sometimes. The goal is to stay consistent, but remember every healthy choice you make counts!

- **Stay Positive:** The journey to managing your blood sugar isn't always easy, but with the right mindset, you can succeed. Celebrate your small wins, and keep moving forward with confidence.

This book is designed to be your companion, a resource that makes managing prediabetes easy, enjoyable, and even fun. I'm here to support you on every step of your journey. Together, we'll build a healthier future, one meal at a time.

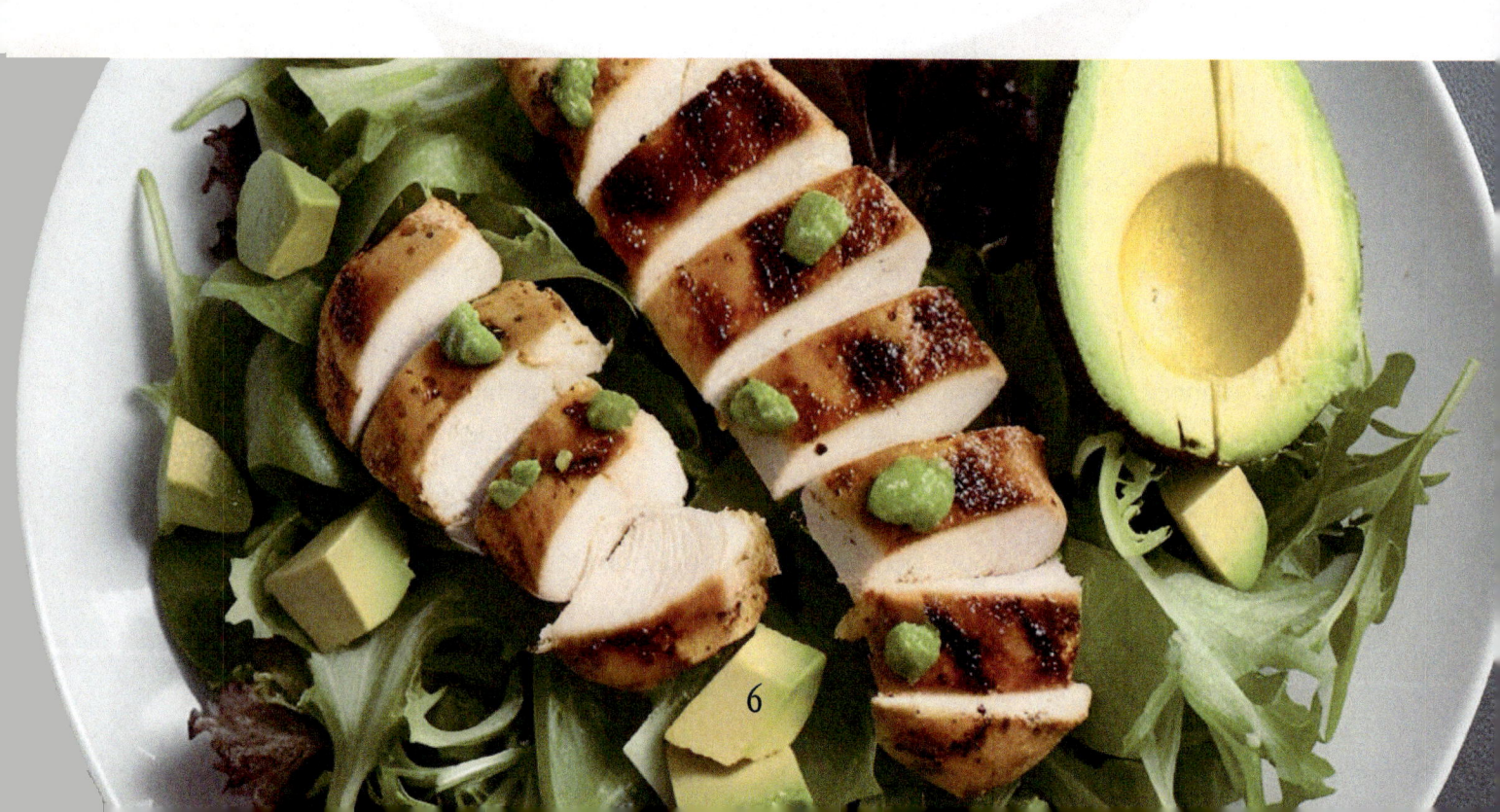

Chapter 1: Foods to Avoid

Managing blood sugar is essential when living with prediabetes, and one of the most impactful ways to do so is by carefully choosing what we eat. Understanding which foods spike your blood sugar and learning how to avoid them can make a world of difference in your health journey. In this chapter, we'll go through the key offenders that contribute to blood sugar spikes and provide simple, healthy alternatives to keep you feeling satisfied without the worry of those spikes.

THE IMPACT OF REFINED CARBS AND SUGARS

Refined carbohydrates and added sugars are two of the biggest culprits when it comes to blood sugar control. These foods are rapidly digested and absorbed by your body, leading to a quick increase in blood sugar levels. Over time, consistently high blood sugar can lead to insulin resistance, where your body becomes less effective at processing glucose, which is a major risk factor for diabetes.

Refined carbohydrates are low in fiber and nutrients. When processed, they lose much of their original nutritional value, leaving behind a product that provides little more than empty calories. Examples of refined carbs include white bread, pastries, cakes, and many breakfast cereals. These foods are often high glycemic, meaning they cause blood sugar to rise quickly.

Added sugars, found in many processed foods like sodas, sugary snacks, and even seemingly harmless foods like yogurts or sauces, can have the same effect. The body doesn't need added sugars for energy, and when consumed in excess, they're stored as fat, leading to increased insulin resistance and higher blood sugar levels.

WHY YOU SHOULD AVOID WHITE BREAD, SUGARY SNACKS, AND SODA

- **White Bread:** Made from refined flour, white bread has very little fiber, which means it lacks the ability to slow down sugar absorption. The result? A quick spike in blood sugar after you eat. Whole grain bread, on the other hand, contains more fiber and slows digestion, helping to maintain more stable blood sugar levels.

- **Sugary Snacks:** It's tempting to reach for a quick, sweet snack when you're hungry, but candy, cookies, and other sugary treats are packed with simple sugars that lead to rapid blood sugar spikes. These snacks also offer little nutritional value, leaving you hungry again soon after eating. Choose snacks like fresh fruit, nuts, or yogurt instead. These alternatives are nutrient-dense and won't cause the same rapid rise in blood sugar.

- **Soda:** Sugary sodas are notorious for causing significant blood sugar spikes. They contain large amounts of added sugars, and their liquid form means they're absorbed into your bloodstream very quickly. Opt for sparkling water, unsweetened iced tea, or even flavored water to satisfy your thirst without all the sugar.

HIGH GLYCEMIC INDEX FOODS TO WATCH OUT FOR

The glycemic index (GI) measures how quickly a food raises your blood sugar levels. High-GI foods are digested and absorbed rapidly, causing a quick surge in blood sugar, which is especially problematic for individuals with prediabetes.
Foods to avoid due to their high glycemic index include:

- **White rice:** Even though it's a staple in many diets, white rice is high in carbohydrates and low in fiber, making it a high-GI food. When possible, substitute it with brown rice, quinoa, or cauliflower rice for a lower-GI, fiber-rich alternative.

- **Pasta:** While pasta is a common comfort food, regular white pasta made from refined flour causes a significant rise in blood sugar. Whole wheat pasta or legume-based pasta (made from chickpeas or lentils) provides more fiber, protein, and a lower glycemic impact.

- **Baked Goods:** Muffins, cookies, and cakes made with refined flour and sugar are not only high in calories but also in glycemic index. Opt for whole grain versions or baking with almond or coconut flour for healthier options.

WHITE RICE, PASTA, AND BAKED GOODS

White Rice: As mentioned earlier, white rice is high in glycemic index. It's processed and stripped of its fiber, which is crucial for slow sugar absorption. Swap white rice for brown rice, wild rice, or quinoa. These grains are higher in fiber, which helps stabilize blood sugar levels.

Pasta: Traditional white pasta can also lead to rapid blood sugar spikes. Instead, choose whole wheat pasta or try spiralized vegetables (like zucchini noodles) for a low-carb, fiber-packed alternative. If you prefer a gluten-free option, chickpea pasta offers a high-protein, lower-GI option.

Baked Goods: Traditional baked goods made from white flour are high in refined sugars and fats. Instead, try using almond flour, coconut flour, or oat flour for a healthier, fiber-rich alternative. You can also use stevia or monk fruit as natural sweeteners instead of refined sugars.

UNHEALTHY FATS: WHAT TO STAY AWAY FROM

When it comes to fats, not all fats are created equal. Some fats, like trans fats and saturated fats, can negatively impact your blood sugar control and increase inflammation, while healthier fats can help manage blood sugar levels and promote overall heart health

TRANS FATS AND PROCESSED MEATS

Trans Fats: These fats are commonly found in fried foods, baked goods, and margarine. Trans fats raise bad cholesterol (LDL) and lower good cholesterol (HDL), which can lead to increased insulin resistance and higher blood sugar levels. Always check the labels and avoid foods containing partially hydrogenated oils. Instead, cook with olive oil or avocado oil, both of which contain heart-healthy monounsaturated fats.

Processed Meats: Meats like bacon, sausages, and hot dogs are not only high in unhealthy fats but also in sodium, which can contribute to high blood pressure. These foods can exacerbate blood sugar control issues. Opt for lean proteins like chicken, turkey, tofu, or fish instead

SUBSTITUTES TO MAKE HEALTHIER CHOICES

The great news is that you don't have to feel deprived when avoiding these foods. There are plenty of substitutions that can help you maintain a satisfying, delicious diet without the blood sugar spikes. Here are some healthy swaps you can easily incorporate into your meals:

- **Substituting White Bread for Whole Grain Bread:** Whole grain bread is a much healthier option because it's made from the entire grain, preserving the fiber, vitamins, and minerals. It has a lower glycemic index and will keep you fuller for longer. Look for bread labeled as 100% whole grain or whole wheat.
- **Using Stevia or Monk Fruit Instead of Sugar:** These natural sweeteners have zero calories and do not spike blood sugar. They're perfect for replacing sugar in baking, beverages, and even desserts.
- **Choosing Avocados Over Mayonnaise:** While mayonnaise is often packed with unhealthy fats, avocados provide healthy fats and fiber. Use mashed avocado as a spread on sandwiches, or mix it into salads for a creamy, nutritious boost.

Managing your blood sugar through a diet doesn't mean giving up your favorite foods. By being mindful of what you eat and making simple substitutions, you can enjoy a variety of tasty, healthy meals that will help stabilize your blood sugar levels and improve your overall health. It's all about making small, sustainable changes that add up to big results.

Chapter 2: Breakfast (A Fresh Start to Your Day)

Starting your day with a balanced breakfast is one of the most effective ways to set yourself up for success, especially when managing prediabetes. The right breakfast can help maintain stable blood sugar levels, provide lasting energy, and even curb unnecessary cravings later in the day. By focusing on high-quality nutrients, fiber, and healthy fats, you can begin each morning with a meal that nourishes both your body and your blood sugar levels.

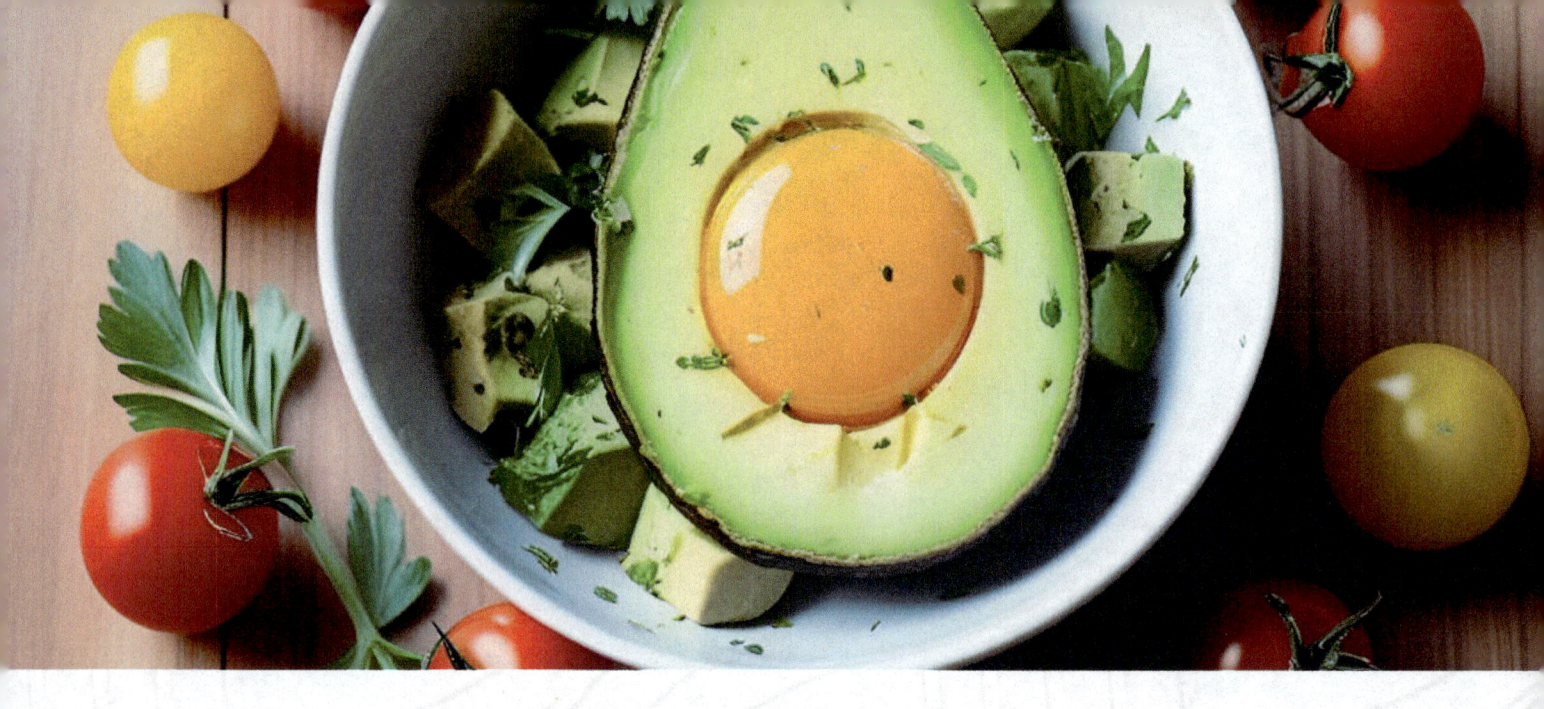

Avocado and Egg Breakfast Bowl

- Prep Time: 5 minutes
- Cook Time: 5 minutes
- Total Time: 10 minutes
- Servings: 1

INGREDIENTS :

- 1 ripe avocado
- 2 large eggs
- 1/4 cup cherry tomatoes, halved
- 1/4 cup spinach (fresh or sautéed)
- 1 tbsp olive oil (for cooking)
- Salt and pepper, to taste

NUTRITIONAL BREAKDOWN (PER SERVING):

- Calories: 300
- Carbs: 14g (5% of daily value)
- Protein: 14g (28% of daily value)
- Fiber: 9g (36% of daily value)
- Fats: 24g (37% of daily value)

HOW TO MAKE :

1. Heat olive oil in a non-stick pan over medium heat.
2. Crack the eggs into the pan and cook them to your desired level of doneness (sunny-side-up, scrambled, or poached).
3. While the eggs are cooking, slice the avocado in half and remove the pit. Scoop out the flesh and slice it.
4. Once the eggs are ready, place them in a bowl. Top with avocado slices, cherry tomatoes, and spinach.
5. Season with a pinch of salt and pepper and drizzle with a bit of olive oil for added flavor and healthy fat.

Oatmeal with Chia Seeds and Berries

- Prep Time: 5 minutes
- Cook Time: 10 minutes
- Total Time: 15 minutes
- Servings: 1

INGREDIENTS :

- 1/2 cup rolled oats (gluten-free if needed)
- 1 cup unsweetened almond milk (or any milk of choice)
- 1 tbsp chia seeds
- 1/4 cup mixed berries (blueberries, raspberries, strawberries)
- 1 tsp cinnamon
- 1 tsp honey or stevia (optional)

NUTRITIONAL BREAKDOWN (PER SERVING):

- Calories: 250
- Carbs: 37g (12% of daily value)
- Protein: 6g (12% of daily value)
- Fiber: 10g (40% of daily value)
- Fats: 9g (14% of daily value)

HOW TO MAKE :

1. In a saucepan, bring almond milk to a simmer over medium heat.
2. Add the oats and cook, stirring occasionally, until the oats are tender and have absorbed most of the liquid (about 5-7 minutes).
3. Stir in chia seeds and cinnamon. Cook for another 2 minutes.
4. Remove from heat and transfer to a bowl.
5. Top with fresh berries and a drizzle of honey or stevia, if desired.

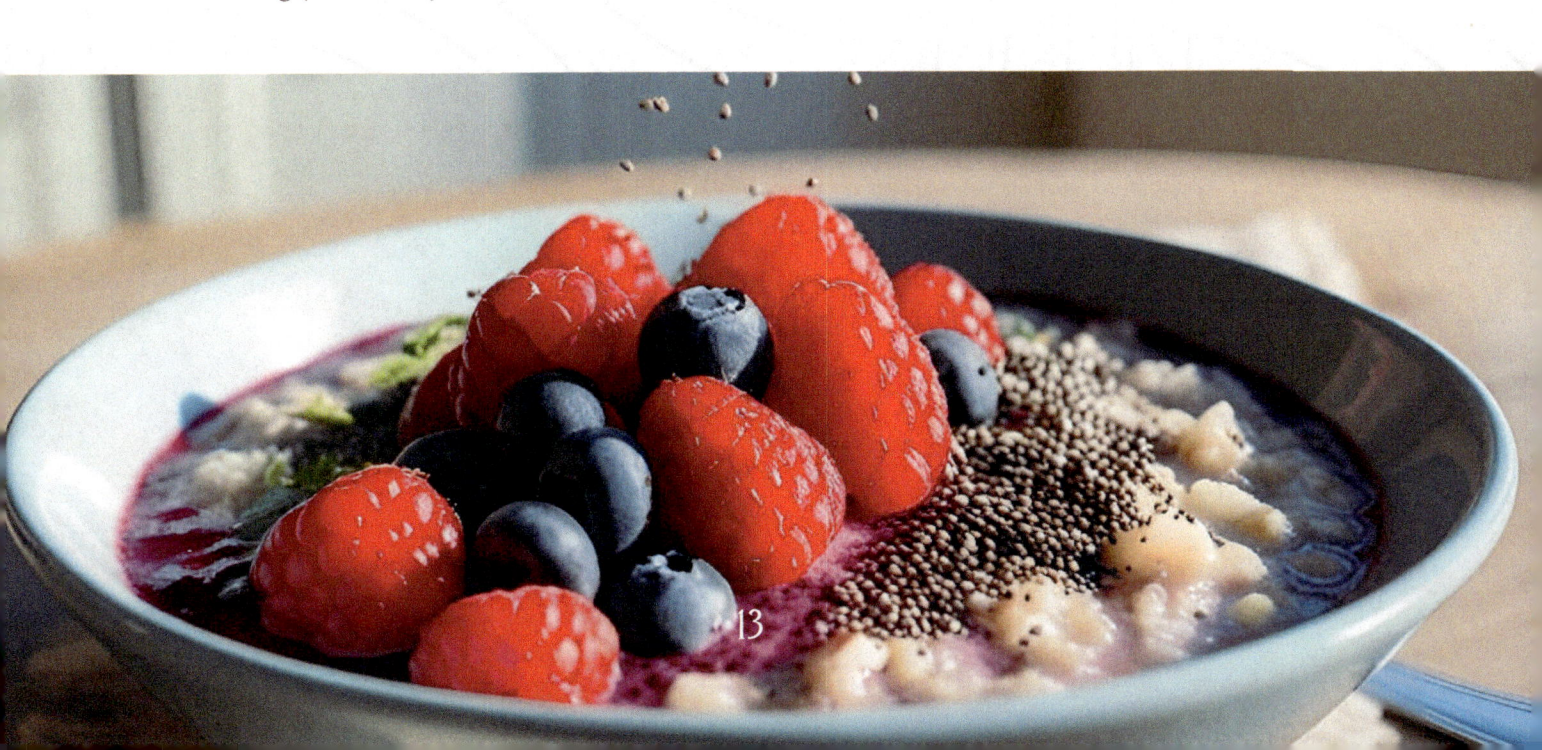

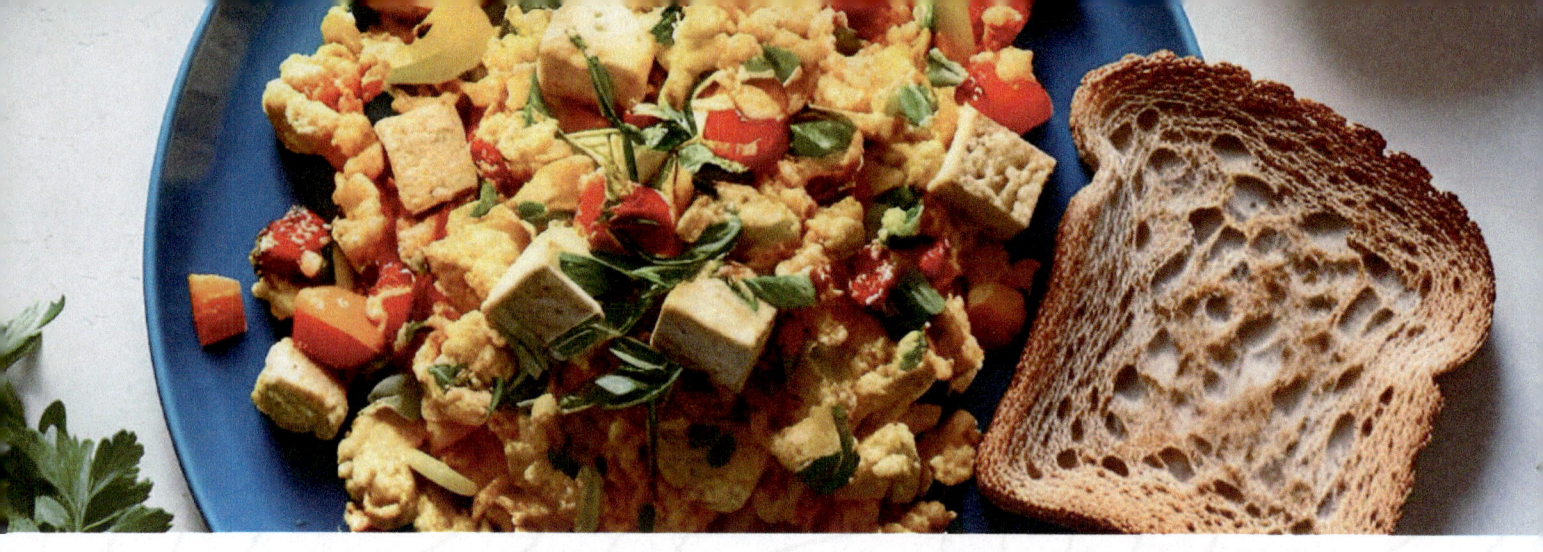

Scrambled Tofu with Veggies and Whole-Grain Toast

- Prep Time: 5 minutes
- Cook Time: 10 minutes
- Total Time: 15 minutes
- Servings: 1

INGREDIENTS :

- 1/2 block firm tofu, crumbled
- 1 tbsp olive oil
- 1/4 cup bell peppers, chopped
- 1/4 cup onions, chopped
- 1/4 cup spinach, chopped
- 1/2 tsp turmeric
- Salt and pepper, to taste
- 1 slice whole-grain toast

HOW TO MAKE :

1. Heat olive oil in a pan over medium heat.
2. Add the bell peppers and onions, sautéing until soft (about 3-4 minutes).
3. Add the crumbled tofu and cook for 5-6 minutes, stirring occasionally.
4. Stir in spinach and turmeric, cooking until the spinach wilts (about 2 minutes).
5. Season with salt and pepper and serve with a slice of toasted whole-grain bread.

NUTRITIONAL BREAKDOWN (PER SERVING):

- Calories: 350
- Carbs: 30g (10% of daily value)
- Protein: 22g (44% of daily value)
- Fiber: 6g (24% of daily value)
- Fats: 20g (31% of daily value)

Almond Butter and Banana Smoothie

- Prep Time: 5 minutes
- Cook Time: None
- Total Time: 5 minutes
- Servings: 1

INGREDIENTS :

- 1 medium banana
- 1 tbsp almond butter
- 1/2 cup unsweetened almond milk
- 1/2 cup spinach (optional for extra greens)
- 1/4 cup Greek yogurt (plain, unsweetened)
- Ice cubes (optional)

HOW TO MAKE :

1. Place all ingredients into a blender and blend until smooth.
2. Add ice cubes for a thicker consistency, if desired.
3. Pour into a glass and enjoy!

NUTRITIONAL BREAKDOWN (PER SERVING):

- Calories: 300
- Carbs: 30g (10% of daily value)
- Protein: 12g (24% of daily value)
- Fiber: 6g (24% of daily value)
- Fats: 17g (26% of daily value)

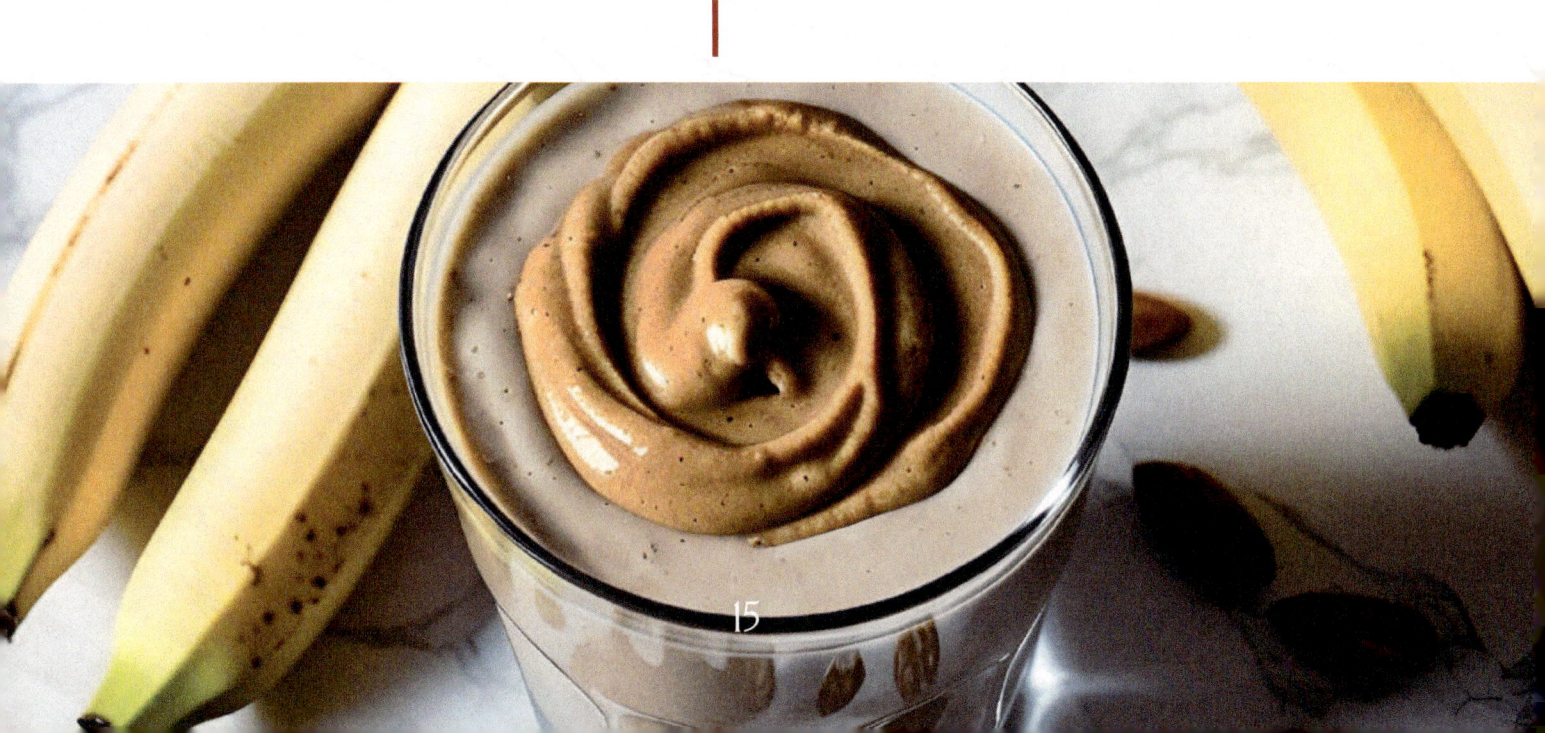

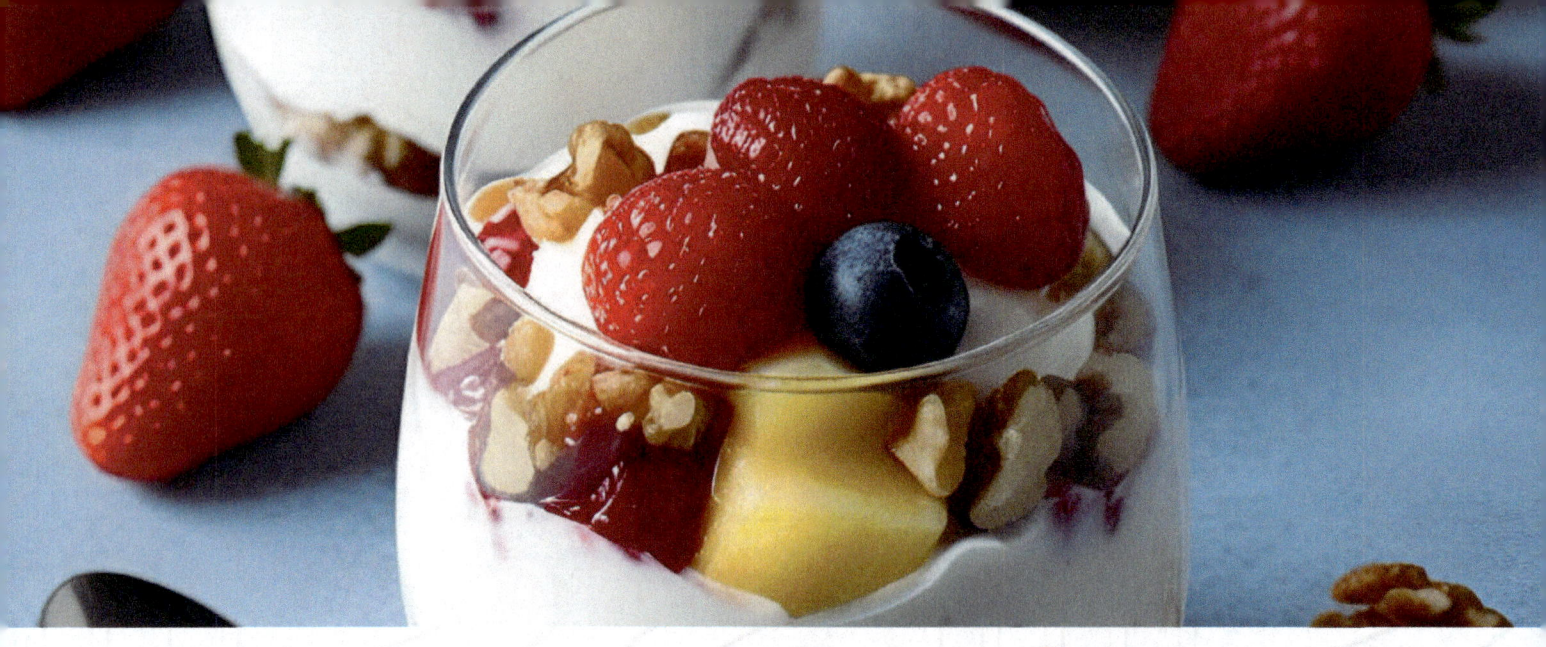

Greek Yogurt Parfait with Fresh Fruit and Walnuts

- Prep Time: 5 minutes
- Cook Time: None
- Total Time: 5 minutes
- Servings: 2

INGREDIENTS :

- 1 cup Greek yogurt (unsweetened)
- 1/4 cup fresh strawberries, sliced
- 1/4 cup blueberries
- 1/4 cup walnuts, chopped
- 1 tsp chia seeds (optional)
- 1 tbsp honey (optional, for sweetness)

NUTRITIONAL BREAKDOWN (PER SERVING):

- Calories: 300
- Carbs: 28g (9% of daily value)
- Protein: 18g (36% of daily value)
- Fiber: 6g (24% of daily value)
- Fats: 18g (28% of daily value)

HOW TO MAKE :

1. In two bowls or jars, layer the Greek yogurt with the fresh strawberries, blueberries, and chopped walnuts.
2. Sprinkle chia seeds over the top if using, and drizzle with a small amount of honey if desired.
3. Serve immediately as a refreshing and satisfying breakfast.

Whole Wheat Pancakes with Blueberry Compote

- Prep Time: 10 minutes
- Cook Time: 15 minutes
- Total Time: 25 minutes
- Servings: 2

INGREDIENTS :

- 1 cup whole wheat flour
- 1/2 tsp baking powder
- 1/4 tsp cinnamon
- 1 egg
- 1/2 cup almond milk (unsweetened)
- 1 tsp vanilla extract
- 1/4 cup fresh blueberries
- 1 tsp honey (optional)
- 1 tbsp olive oil (for cooking)

NUTRITIONAL BREAKDOWN (PER SERVING):

- Calories: 350
- Carbs: 50g (17% of daily value)
- Protein: 8g (16% of daily value)
- Fiber: 8g (32% of daily value)
- Fats: 10g (15% of daily value)

HOW TO MAKE :

1. In a bowl, whisk together the whole wheat flour, baking powder, cinnamon, egg, almond milk, and vanilla extract to make the pancake batter.
2. Heat a skillet or griddle over medium heat and lightly grease it with olive oil.
3. Pour the batter onto the skillet in small circles and cook for 2-3 minutes per side, until golden brown.
4. For the blueberry compote: In a small saucepan, heat the fresh blueberries with honey (if using) over low heat for 3-4 minutes until the berries soften and release their juices.
5. Serve the pancakes with the blueberry compote drizzled over the top.

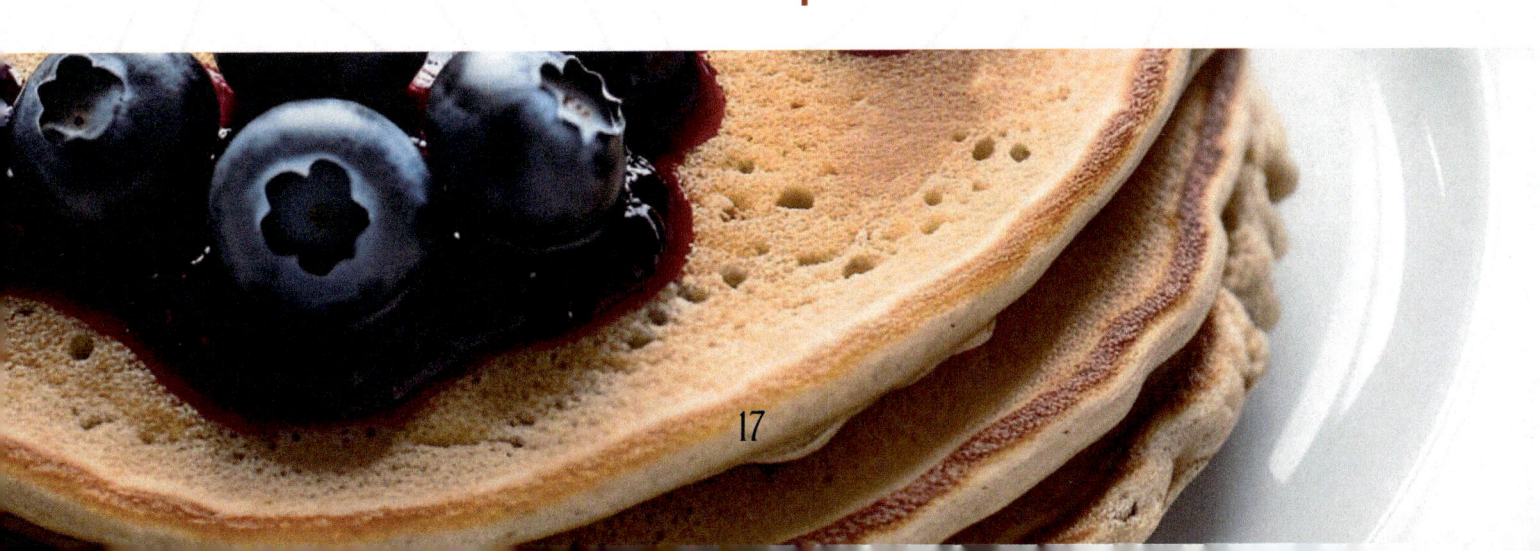

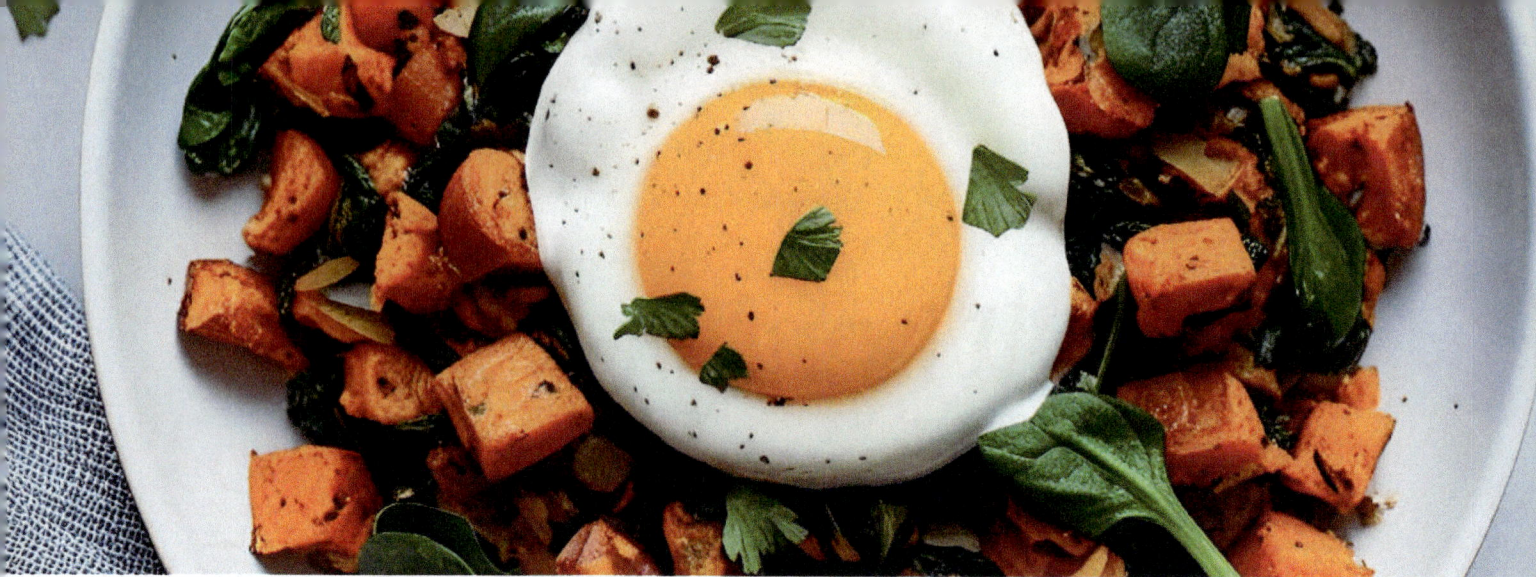

Sweet Potato and Spinach Breakfast Hash

- Prep Time: 10 minutes
- Cook Time: 20 minutes
- Total Time: 30 minutes
- Servings: 2

INGREDIENTS :

- 1 medium sweet potato, peeled and diced
- 1 tbsp olive oil
- 1/2 cup onion, chopped
- 1 cup spinach, chopped
- 1/2 tsp cumin
- Salt and pepper, to taste
- 1/2 avocado, diced (optional, for topping)

NUTRITIONAL BREAKDOWN (PER SERVING):

- Calories: 350
- Carbs: 45g (15% of daily value)
- Protein: 6g (12% of daily value)
- Fiber: 10g (40% of daily value)
- Fats: 18g (28% of daily value)

HOW TO MAKE :

1. Heat olive oil in a skillet over medium heat. Add the diced sweet potato and cook for 10-12 minutes, stirring occasionally, until tender and slightly crispy.
2. Add the chopped onion and cook for an additional 3-4 minutes until softened.
3. Stir in the chopped spinach, cumin, salt, and pepper, and cook for another 2-3 minutes, until the spinach wilts.
4. Serve the hash topped with diced avocado for an extra boost of healthy fats.

Quinoa Porridge with Cinnamon and Almonds

- Prep Time: 5 minutes
- Cook Time: 15 minutes
- Total Time: 20 minutes
- Servings: 2

INGREDIENTS :

- 1/2 cup quinoa, rinsed
- 1 cup almond milk (unsweetened)
- 1/4 tsp cinnamon
- 1 tbsp sliced almonds
- 1 tbsp chia seeds (optional)
- 1 tsp honey or stevia (optional)

NUTRITIONAL BREAKDOWN (PER SERVING):

- Calories: 250
- Carbs: 32g (11% of daily value)
- Protein: 7g (14% of daily value)
- Fiber: 6g (24% of daily value)
- Fats: 10g (15% of daily value)

HOW TO MAKE :

1. In a small pot, combine quinoa and almond milk. Bring to a boil, then reduce the heat to low and cover. Cook for 12-15 minutes until the quinoa is tender and the liquid is absorbed.
2. Stir in cinnamon and optional sweetener (honey or stevia), and cook for another 1-2 minutes.
3. Serve topped with sliced almonds and chia seeds for added texture and healthy fats.

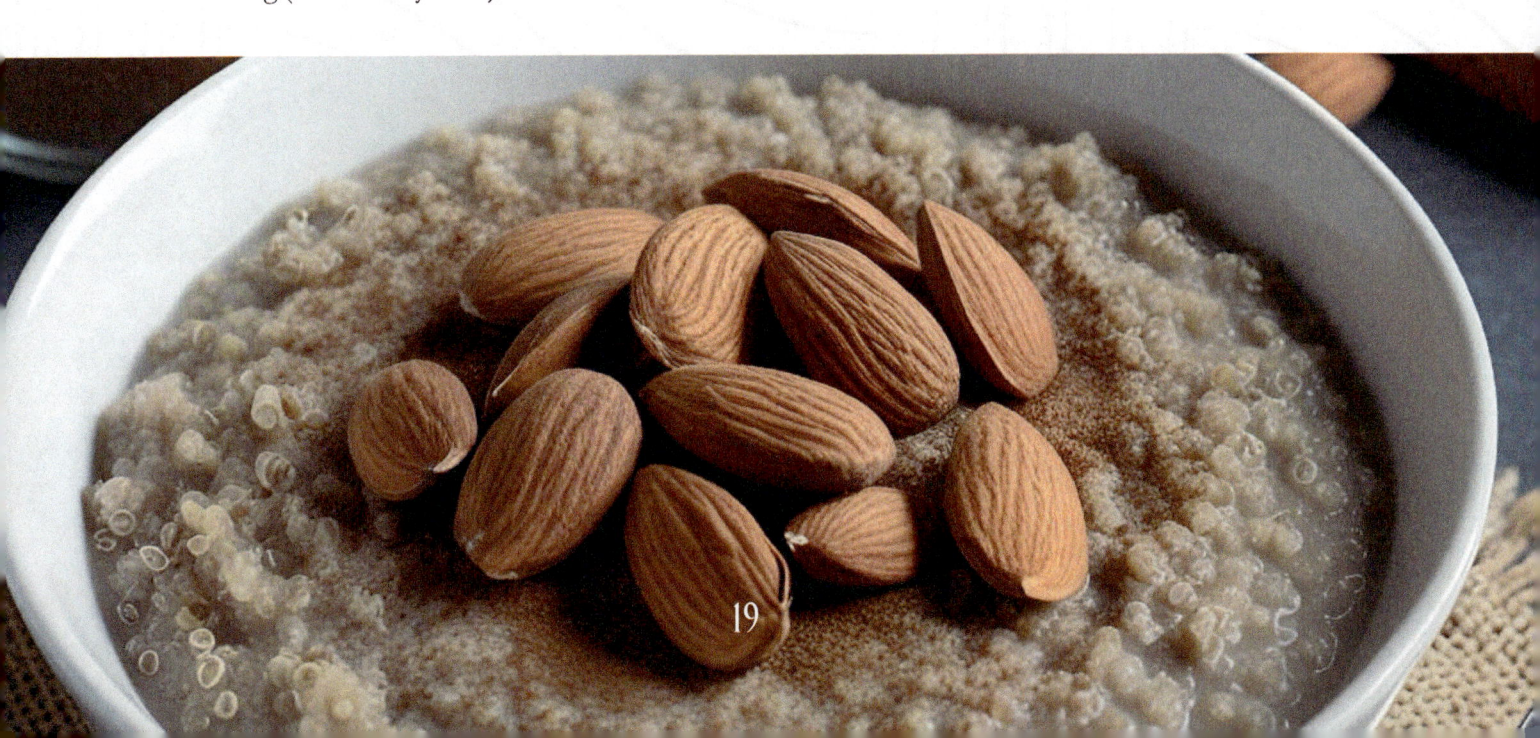

Chapter 3: Lunch
(Keeping Your Energy Stable)

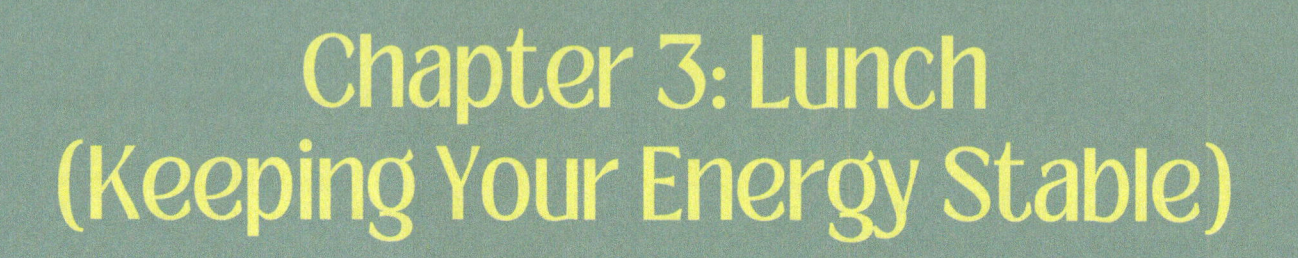

Lunchtime often comes with the challenge of balancing blood sugar while also staying satisfied and energized for the second half of the day. For individuals managing prediabetes, balanced lunches that combine protein, fiber, and healthy fats are essential to stabilize blood sugar and keep energy levels steady. The goal of your lunch should be to avoid the post-lunch slump while helping to control hunger and cravings.

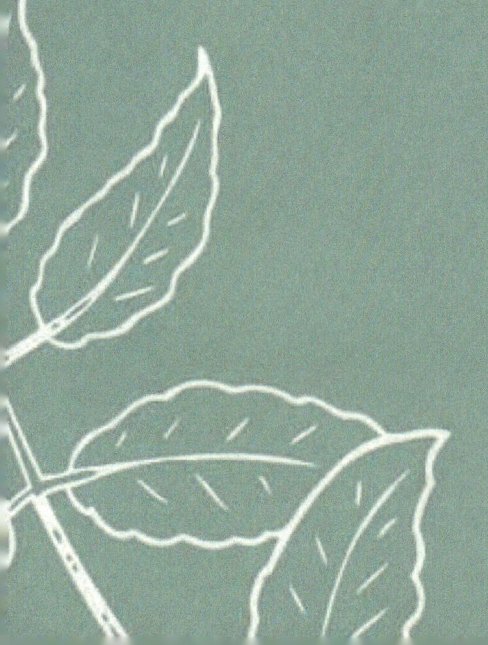

Quinoa and Chickpea Salad with Lemon-Tahini Dressing

- Prep Time: 10 minutes
- Cook Time: 15 minutes
- Total Time: 25 minutes
- Servings: 2

INGREDIENTS :

- 1 cup quinoa (uncooked)
- 1 can (15 oz) chickpeas, drained and rinsed
- 1/2 cucumber, diced
- 1/4 cup red onion, finely chopped
- 1/4 cup fresh parsley, chopped
- 1 tbsp olive oil

FOR LEMON-TAHINI DRESSING:

- 2 tbsp tahini
- 1 tbsp lemon juice
- 1 tsp Dijon mustard
- 1 tbsp olive oil
- 1 tbsp water (to thin)
- Salt and pepper to taste

HOW TO MAKE :

1. Cook quinoa according to package instructions (typically about 15 minutes).
2. In a large bowl, combine the cooked quinoa, chickpeas, cucumber, red onion, and parsley.
3. In a small bowl, whisk together tahini, lemon juice, Dijon mustard, olive oil, and water. Add salt and pepper to taste.
4. Pour the dressing over the salad and toss to coat evenly. Serve chilled or at room temperature.

NUTRITIONAL BREAKDOWN (PER SERVING):

- Calories: 350
- Carbs: 40g (13% of daily value)
- Protein: 12g (24% of daily value)
- Fiber: 10g (40% of daily value)
- Fats: 14g (22% of daily value)

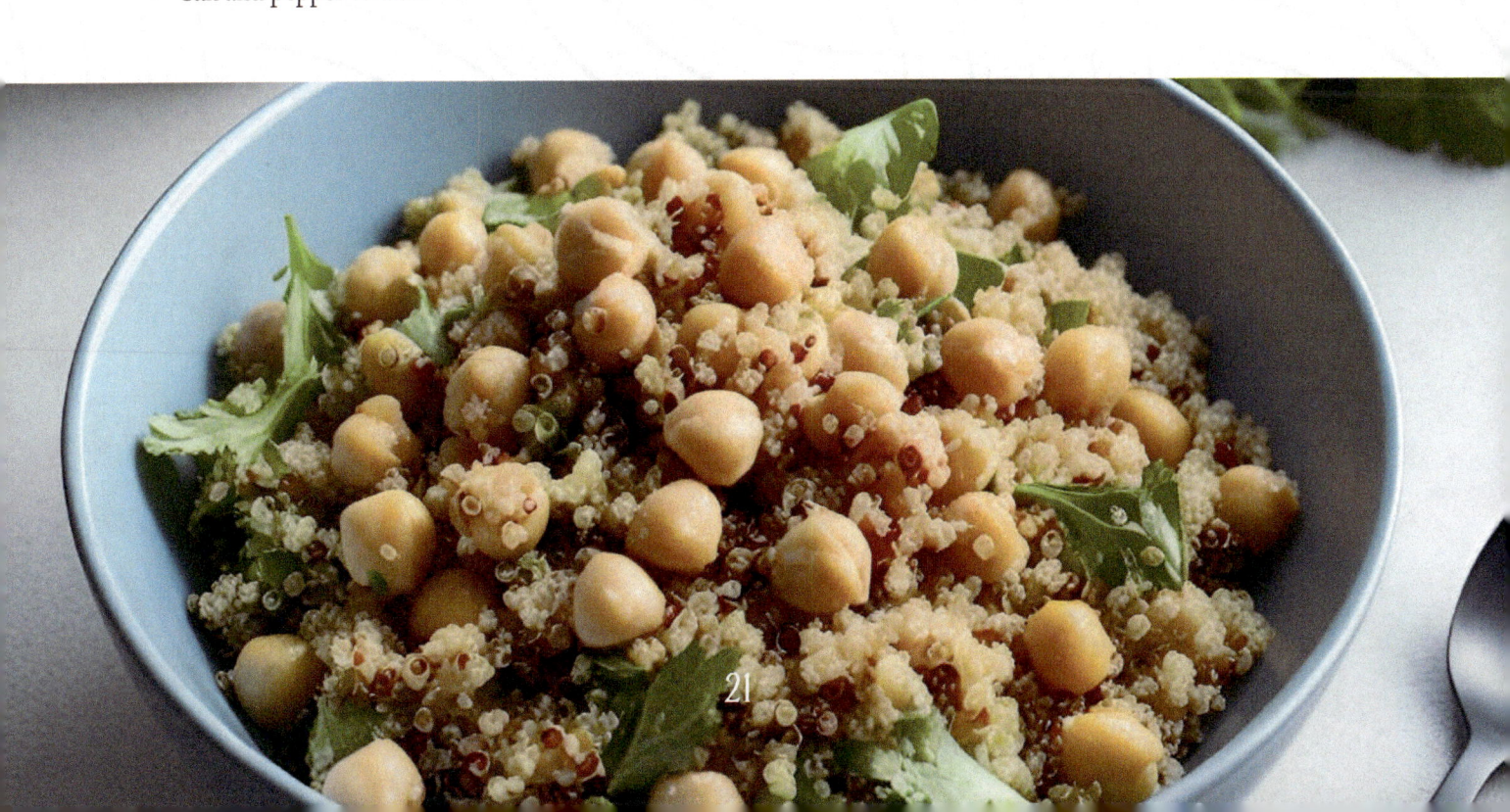

Grilled Chicken and Avocado Salad

- Prep Time: 10 minutes
- Cook Time: 10 minutes
- Total Time: 20 minutes
- Servings: 1

INGREDIENTS :

- 1 boneless, skinless chicken breast
- 1 tsp olive oil
- Salt and pepper, to taste
- 1/2 avocado, sliced
- 2 cups mixed greens (spinach, arugula, or lettuce)
- 1/4 cup cherry tomatoes, halved
- 1/4 cucumber, sliced

FOR LEMON-TAHINI DRESSING:

- 1 tbsp olive oil
- 1 tbsp balsamic vinegar
- 1 tsp Dijon mustard
- Salt and pepper, to taste

HOW TO MAKE :

1. Heat a grill pan or skillet over medium-high heat. Season the chicken breast with olive oil, salt, and pepper.
2. Grill the chicken for about 5-7 minutes per side, until fully cooked and juices run clear. Allow the chicken to rest for a few minutes, then slice thinly.
3. In a bowl, toss the mixed greens, cherry tomatoes, cucumber, and sliced avocado.
4. In a small bowl, whisk together olive oil, balsamic vinegar, Dijon mustard, salt, and pepper for the dressing.
5. Top the salad with grilled chicken and drizzle with dressing.

NUTRITIONAL BREAKDOWN (PER SERVING):

- Calories: 210
- Protein: 3g (6% of daily intake)
- Fat: 16g (24% of daily intake)
- Carbs: 24g (8% of daily intake)
- Fiber: 5g (20% of daily intake)
- Vitamin A: 180% of daily intake (from butternut squash)

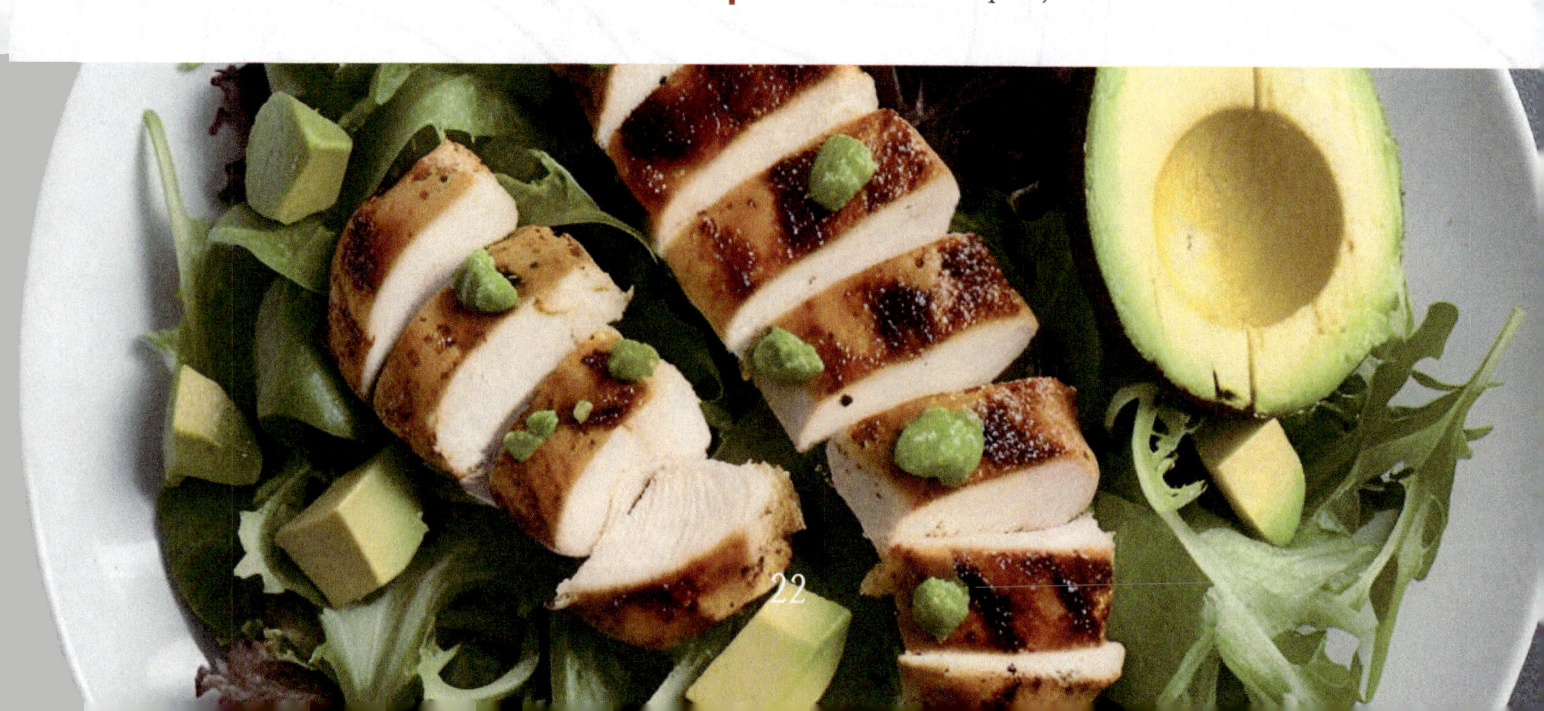

Zucchini Noodles with Pesto and Cherry Tomatoes

- Prep Time: 10 minutes
- Cook Time: 5 minutes
- Total Time: 15 minutes
- Servings: 1

INGREDIENTS :

- 1 medium zucchini, spiralized into noodles
- 1/2 cup cherry tomatoes, halved
- 1/4 cup pesto (store-bought or homemade)
- 1 tbsp olive oil
- 1 tbsp grated Parmesan cheese (optional)

NUTRITIONAL BREAKDOWN (PER SERVING):

- Calories: 220
- Carbs: 12g (4% of daily value)
- Protein: 6g (12% of daily value)
- Fiber: 5g (20% of daily value)
- Fats: 18g (28% of daily value)

HOW TO MAKE :

1. Heat olive oil in a skillet over medium heat. Add zucchini noodles and sauté for 2-3 minutes until just tender.
2. Add the halved cherry tomatoes and cook for another 2 minutes, stirring occasionally.
3. Remove from heat and stir in the pesto sauce, coating the noodles and tomatoes evenly.
4. Top with grated Parmesan, if desired, and serve immediately.

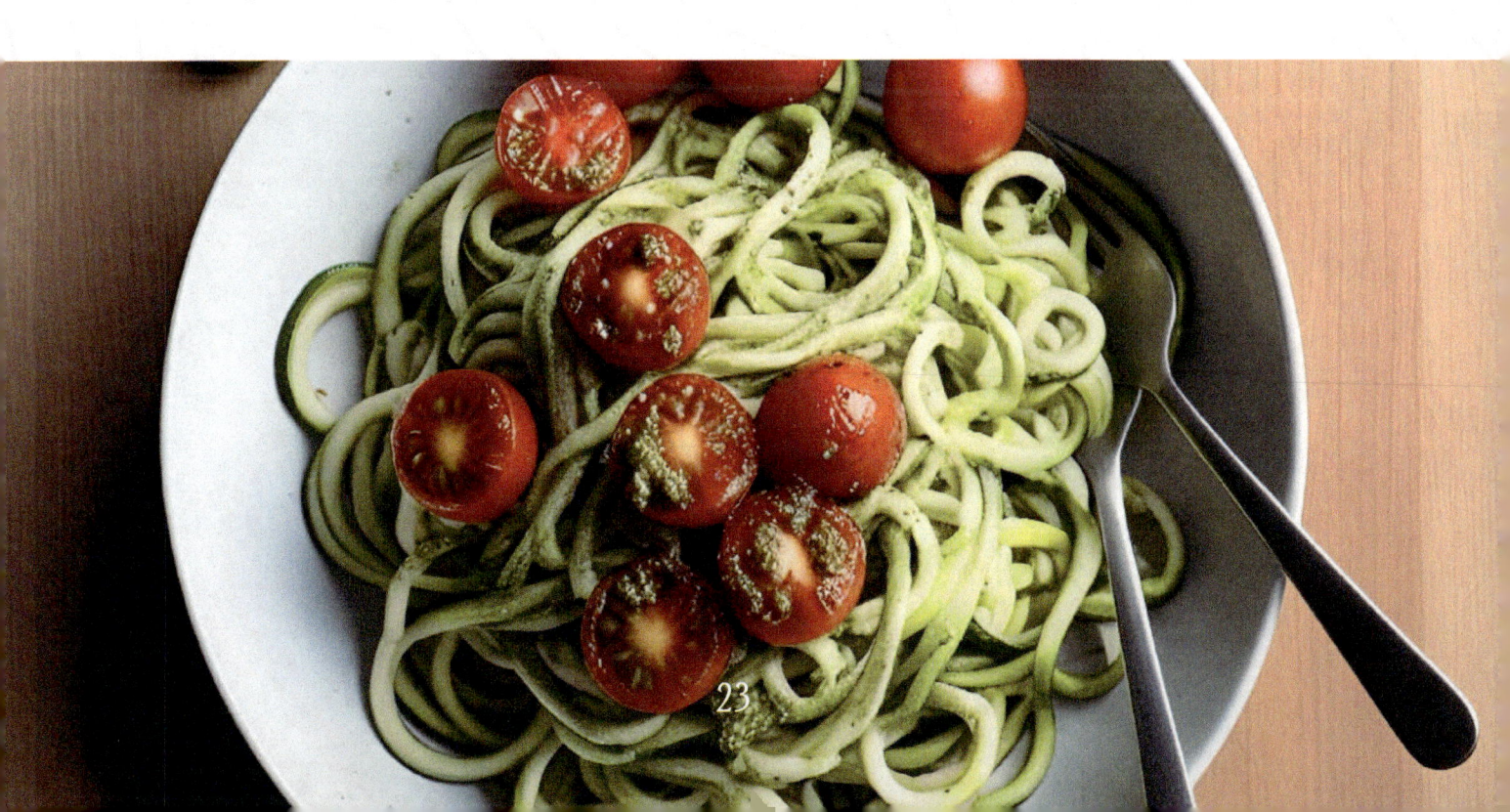

Lentil Soup with Spinach and Carrots

- Prep Time: 10 minutes
- Cook Time: 30 minutes
- Total Time: 40 minutes
- Servings: 4

INGREDIENTS :

- 1 cup dried lentils, rinsed
- 1 tbsp olive oil
- 1 small onion, chopped
- 2 carrots, diced
- 2 garlic cloves, minced
- 4 cups vegetable broth
- 1/2 tsp cumin
- 1/2 tsp paprika
- 2 cups fresh spinach, chopped
- Salt and pepper, to taste

HOW TO MAKE :

1. Heat olive oil in a large pot over medium heat. Add onions and carrots and sauté for about 5 minutes until softened.
2. Add garlic, cumin, and paprika, cooking for another minute until fragrant.
3. Pour in the vegetable broth and bring to a simmer. Add lentils and cook for 25-30 minutes, or until lentils are tender.
4. Stir in the spinach and cook for an additional 2 minutes until wilted.
5. Season with salt and pepper to taste and serve.

NUTRITIONAL BREAKDOWN (PER SERVING):

- Calories: 250
- Carbs: 40g (13% of daily value)
- Protein: 15g (30% of daily value)
- Fiber: 15g (60% of daily value)
- Fats: 6g (9% of daily value)

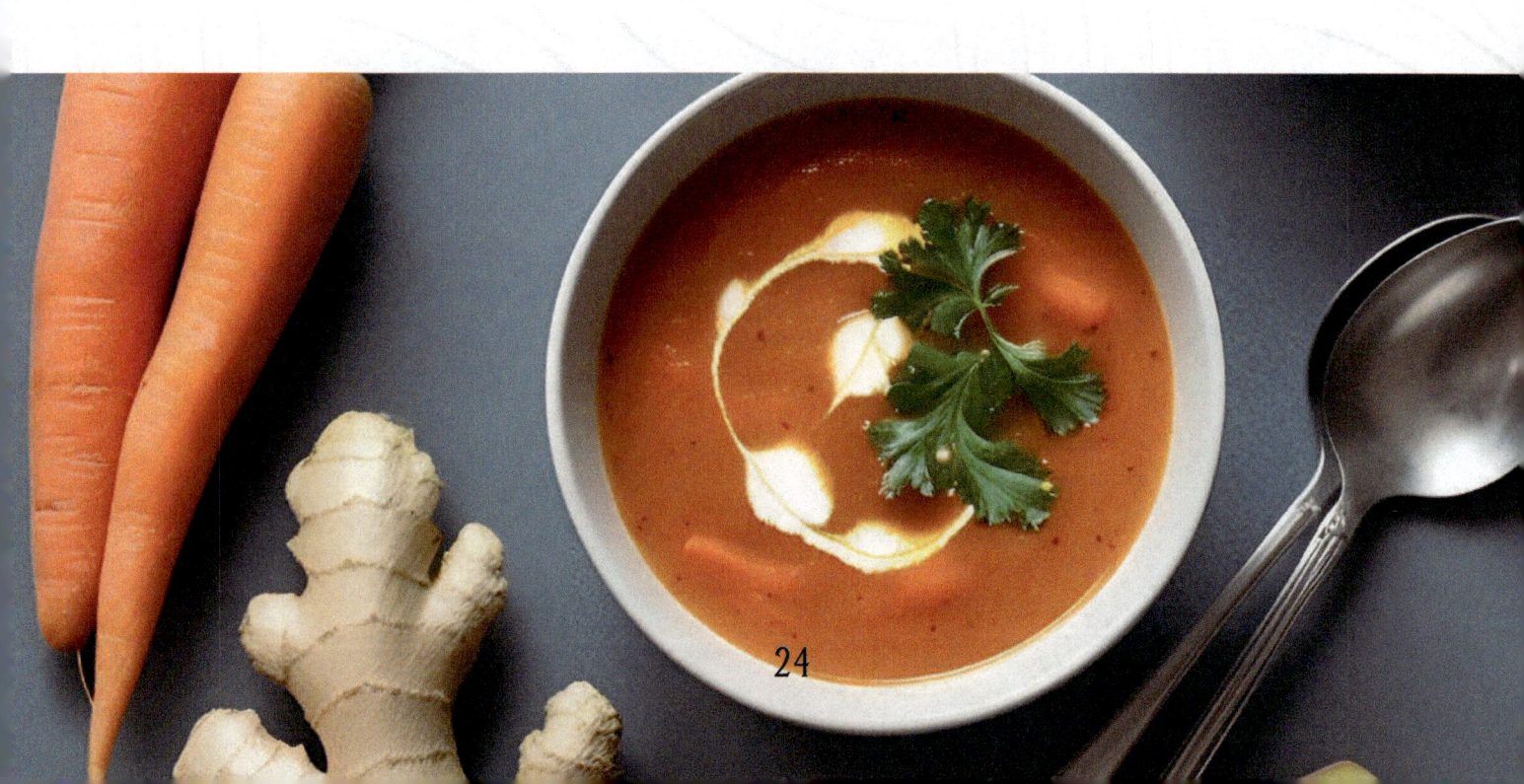

Tuna Salad Lettuce Wraps

- Prep Time: 10 minutes
- Cook Time: None
- Total Time: 10 minutes
- Servings: 2

INGREDIENTS :

- 1 can (5 oz) tuna in water, drained
- 1/4 cup plain Greek yogurt (unsweetened)
- 1 tbsp Dijon mustard
- 1 tbsp lemon juice
- 1/4 cup celery, diced
- 1/4 cup red onion, finely chopped
- Salt and pepper, to taste
- 4 large lettuce leaves (e.g., Romaine or Butter lettuce)

HOW TO MAKE :

1. In a bowl, combine the tuna, Greek yogurt, Dijon mustard, and lemon juice.
2. Add diced celery, red onion, and season with salt and pepper to taste. Mix everything together until well combined.
3. Spoon the tuna salad into the center of each lettuce leaf.
4. Wrap the lettuce around the filling like a taco and enjoy!

NUTRITIONAL BREAKDOWN (PER SERVING):

- Calories: 250
- Carbs: 5g (2% of daily value)
- Protein: 30g (60% of daily value)
- Fiber: 2g (8% of daily value)
- Fats: 14g (22% of daily value)

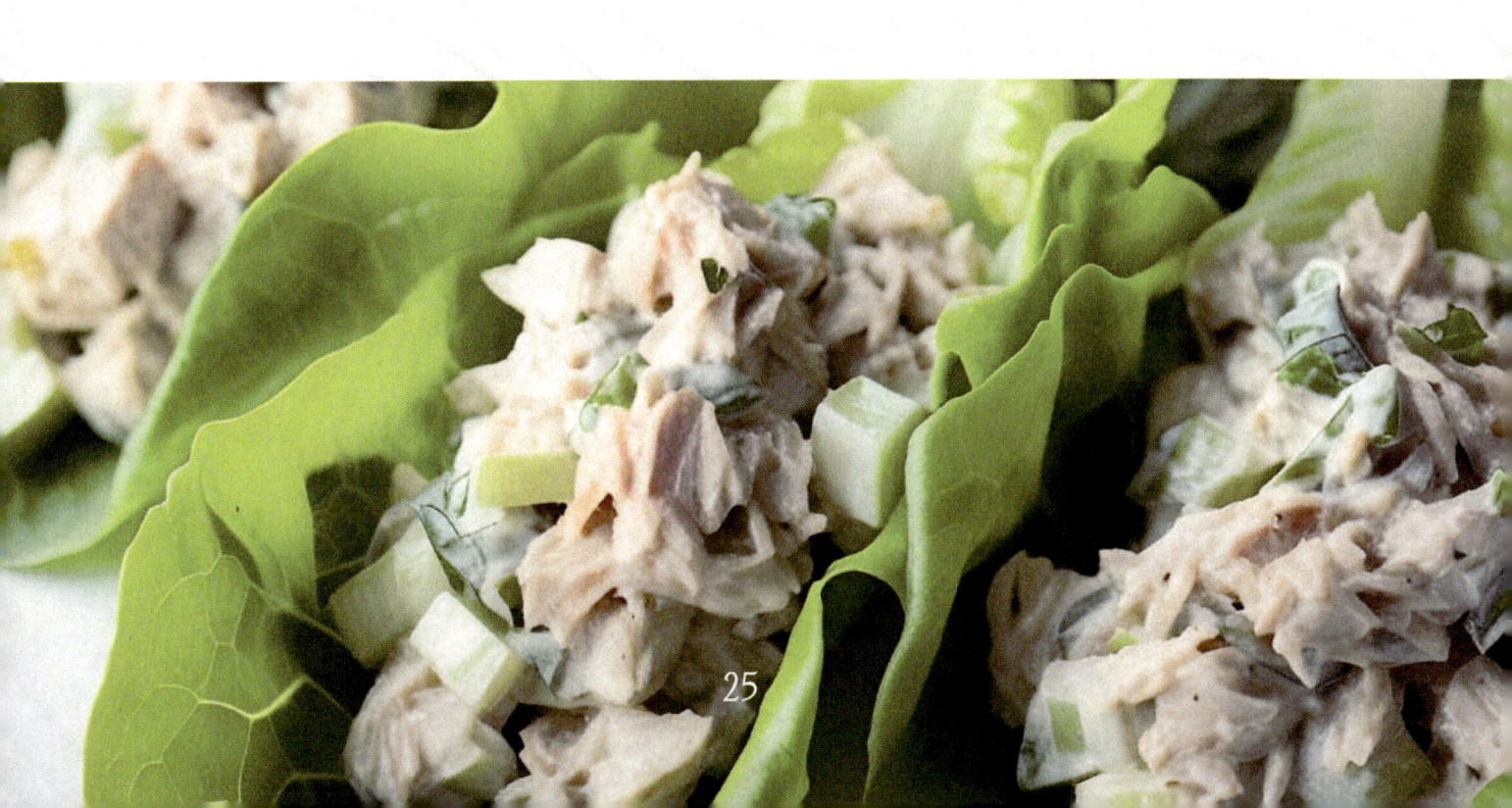

Sweet Potato and Black Bean Tacos

- Prep Time: 10 minutes
- Cook Time: 15 minutes
- Total Time: 25 minutes
- Servings: 2

INGREDIENTS :

- 1 medium sweet potato, peeled and diced
- 1 tsp olive oil
- 1/2 tsp cumin
- 1/2 tsp chili powder
- 1/2 tsp paprika
- 1 can (15 oz) black beans, drained and rinsed
- 4 small corn tortillas
- 1/4 cup fresh cilantro, chopped
- 1/4 cup red onion, finely chopped
- 1/4 cup salsa (optional)
- Lime wedges, for serving

HOW TO MAKE :

1. Preheat your oven to 400°F (200°C).
2. Toss the diced sweet potato with olive oil, cumin, chili powder, and paprika. Spread the sweet potatoes on a baking sheet and roast for 15 minutes, or until tender and slightly crispy.
3. While the sweet potatoes roast, warm the black beans in a small pot over medium heat.
4. Once the sweet potatoes are ready, assemble the tacos: layer each corn tortilla with black beans, roasted sweet potato, chopped cilantro, and red onion.
5. Top with salsa and a squeeze of lime, if desired, and enjoy!

NUTRITIONAL BREAKDOWN (PER SERVING):

- Calories: 350
- Carbs: 55g (18% of daily value)
- Protein: 10g (20% of daily value)
- Fiber: 14g (56% of daily value)
- Fats: 10g (15% of daily value)

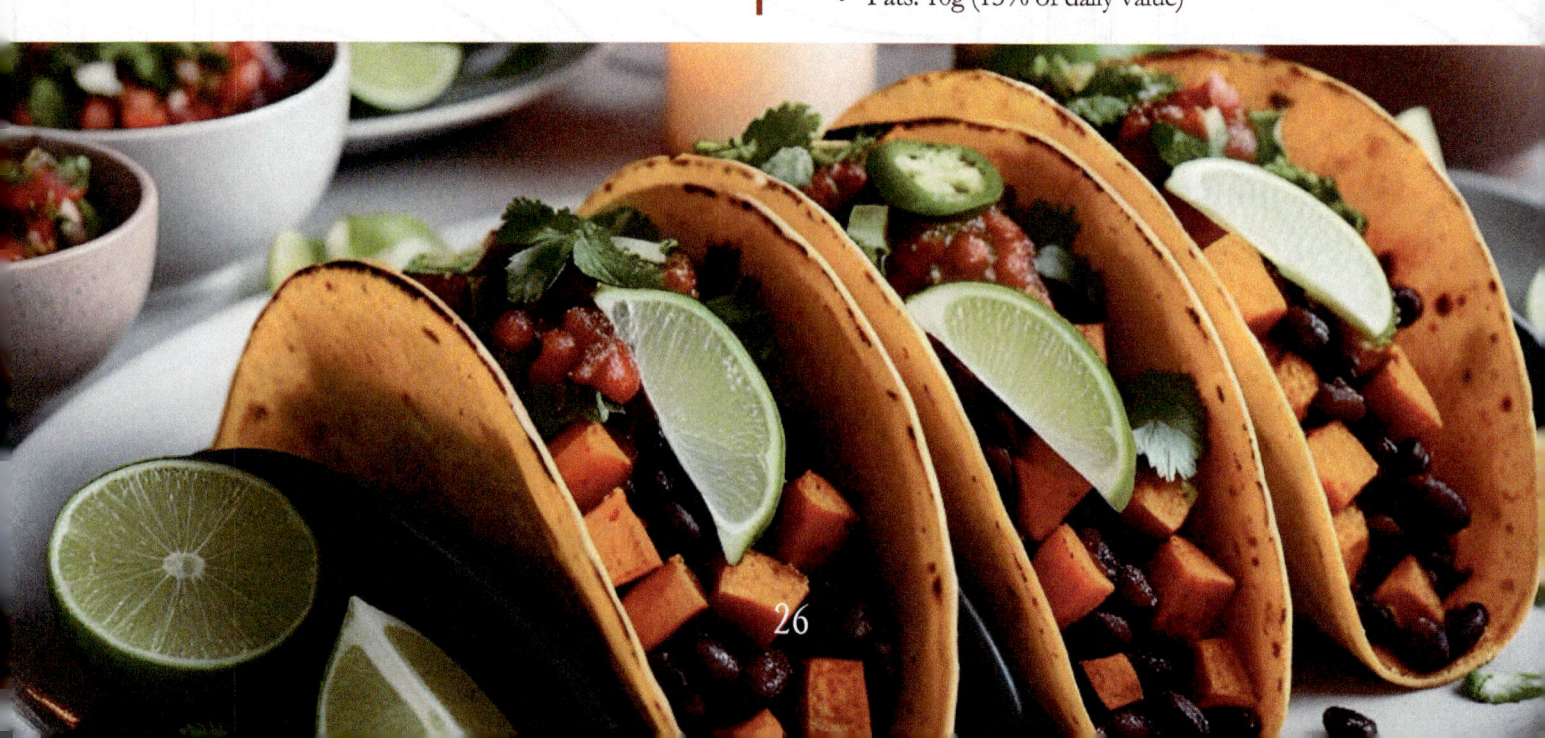

Veggie-Stuffed Whole Wheat Pita with Hummus

- Prep Time: 10 minutes
- Cook Time: None
- Total Time: 10 minutes
- Servings: 1

INGREDIENTS :

- 1 whole wheat pita
- 1/4 cup hummus (store-bought or homemade)
- 1/4 cucumber, thinly sliced
- 1/4 cup shredded carrots
- 1/4 cup bell pepper, thinly sliced
- 1/4 cup spinach or mixed greens
- 1 tbsp olive oil (optional, for drizzling)
- Salt and pepper, to taste

HOW TO MAKE :

1. Cut the whole wheat pita in half to create two pockets.
2. Spread hummus inside each pita half.
3. Layer in the cucumber, carrots, bell pepper, and spinach or mixed greens.
4.
5. Drizzle with olive oil (if desired) and season with salt and pepper.
6. Serve immediately or wrap it up for a quick lunch on the go.

NUTRITIONAL BREAKDOWN (PER SERVING):

- Calories: 300
- Carbs: 35g (12% of daily value)
- Protein: 9g (18% of daily value)
- Fiber: 10g (40% of daily value)
- Fats: 14g (22% of daily value)

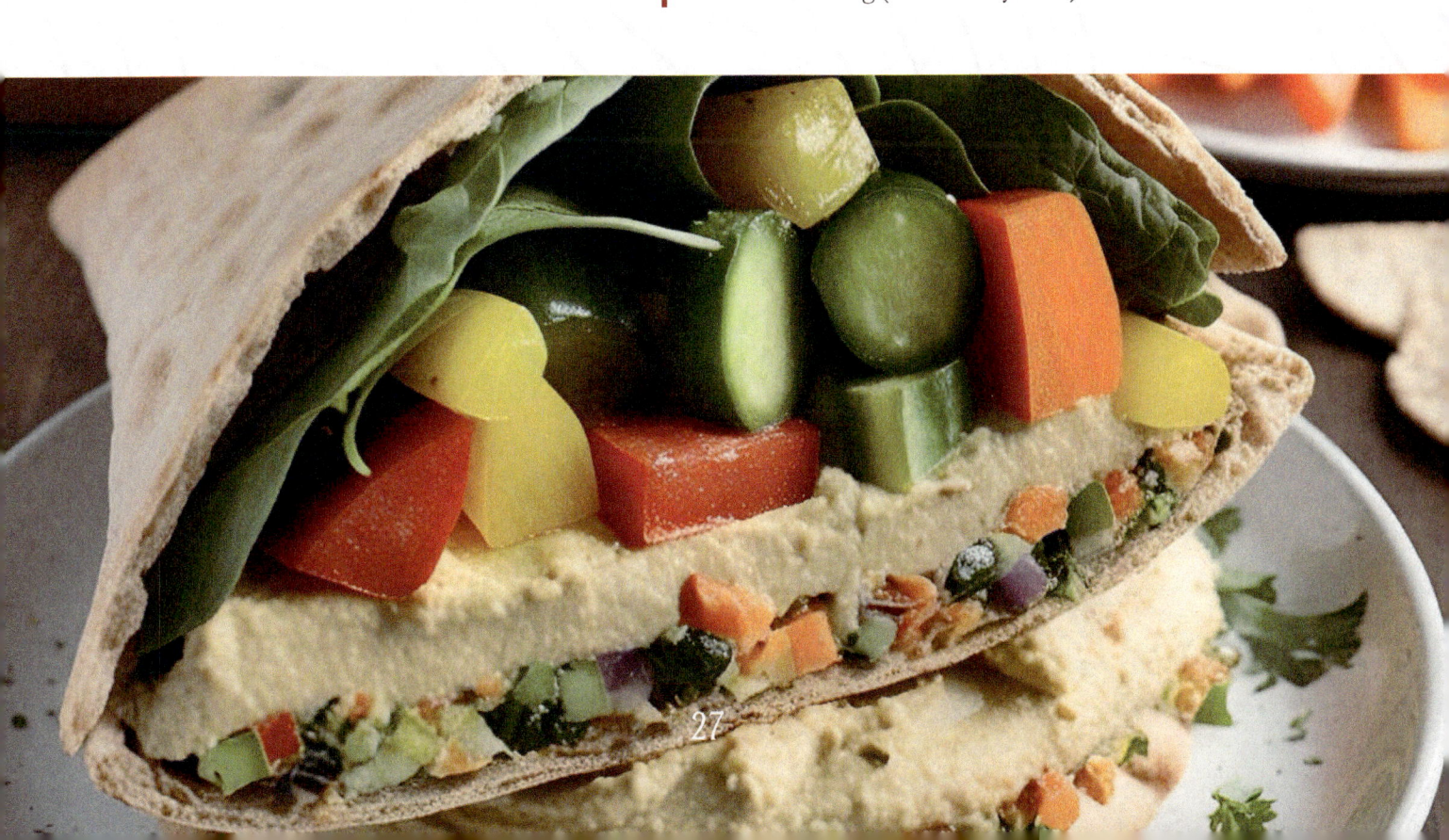

Baked Salmon with Roasted Veggies

- Prep Time: 10 minutes
- Cook Time: 20 minutes
- Total Time: 30 minutes
- Servings: 2

INGREDIENTS :

- 2 salmon fillets (4 oz each)
- 1 tbsp olive oil
- 1 tsp lemon zest
- 1/2 tsp garlic powder
- Salt and pepper, to taste
- 1 cup broccoli florets
- 1 medium sweet potato, diced
- 1/2 red onion, sliced
- 1 tbsp fresh parsley, chopped (optional)

NUTRITIONAL BREAKDOWN (PER SERVING):

- Calories: 400
- Carbs: 30g (10% of daily value)
- Protein: 30g (60% of daily value)
- Fiber: 8g (32% of daily value)
- Fats: 20g (31% of daily value)

HOW TO MAKE :

1. Preheat your oven to 400°F (200°C).
2. Place the salmon fillets on a baking sheet lined with parchment paper. Drizzle with olive oil, lemon zest, garlic powder, salt, and pepper.
3. On the same baking sheet, toss the broccoli, sweet potato, and red onion with olive oil, salt, and pepper. Spread them out in a single layer.
4. Roast everything in the oven for 18-20 minutes, or until the salmon is cooked through and flakes easily with a fork. The vegetables should be tender and slightly browned.
5. Serve the salmon with the roasted veggies and top with fresh parsley.

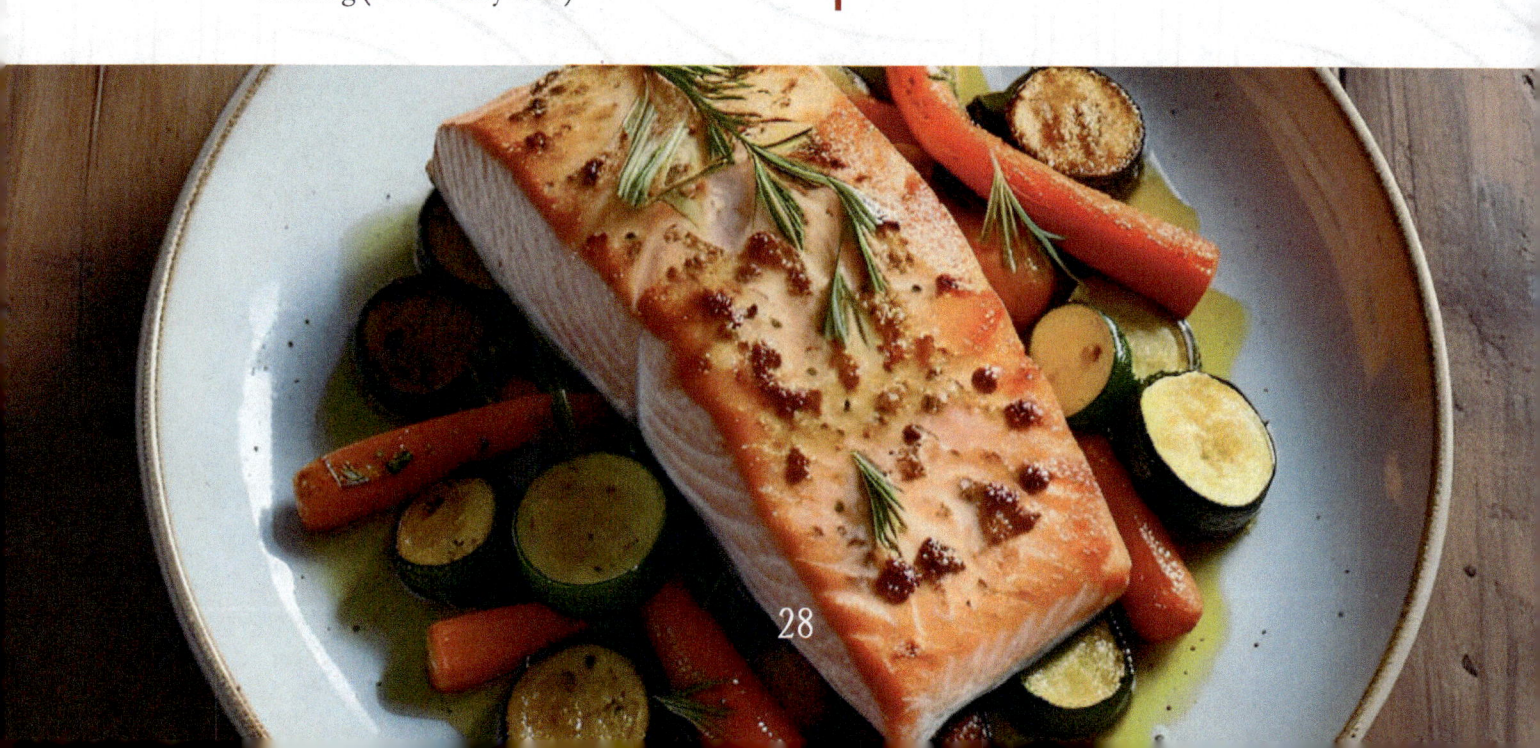

Chapter 4: Dinner (Nourishing Your Body and Soul)

As the day comes to a close, dinner offers the perfect opportunity to nourish your body with wholesome, satisfying meals that support your health goals. When managing prediabetes, it's important to focus on meals that are both heart-healthy and blood sugar-friendly. Dinner should be a time to wind down and treat yourself to delicious, balanced meals that leave you feeling nourished, not sluggish.

A well-rounded dinner should include a combination of protein, fiber, and healthy fats to stabilize blood sugar, promote satiety, and prevent cravings. However, it's important to practice portion control to avoid overeating, especially as our bodies are winding down after a long day. Remember, balance is key.

Grilled Chicken with Quinoa and Roasted Broccoli

- Prep Time: 10 minutes
- Cook Time: 20 minutes
- Total Time: 30 minutes
- Servings: 2

INGREDIENTS :

- 2 boneless, skinless chicken breasts
- 1 tsp olive oil
- 1/2 tsp garlic powder
- 1/2 tsp paprika
- Salt and pepper, to taste
- 1 cup quinoa (uncooked)
- 2 cups broccoli florets
- 1 tbsp olive oil (for roasting)
- 1 tbsp lemon juice (optional)

NUTRITIONAL BREAKDOWN (PER SERVING):

- Calories: 450
- Carbs: 35g (12% of daily value)
- Protein: 40g (80% of daily value)
- Fiber: 8g (32% of daily value)
- Fats: 18g (28% of daily value)

HOW TO MAKE :

1. Preheat the grill or a grill pan over medium heat.
2. Rub the chicken breasts with olive oil, garlic powder, paprika, salt, and pepper.
3. Grill the chicken for 5-7 minutes per side, or until fully cooked and the internal temperature reaches 165°F (75°C).
4. Meanwhile, cook quinoa according to package instructions (about 15 minutes).
5. Preheat the oven to 400°F (200°C). Toss the broccoli florets with olive oil, salt, and pepper, and roast on a baking sheet for 15 minutes, flipping halfway through
6. Serve the grilled chicken alongside quinoa and roasted broccoli. Drizzle with lemon juice for a fresh, zesty finish.

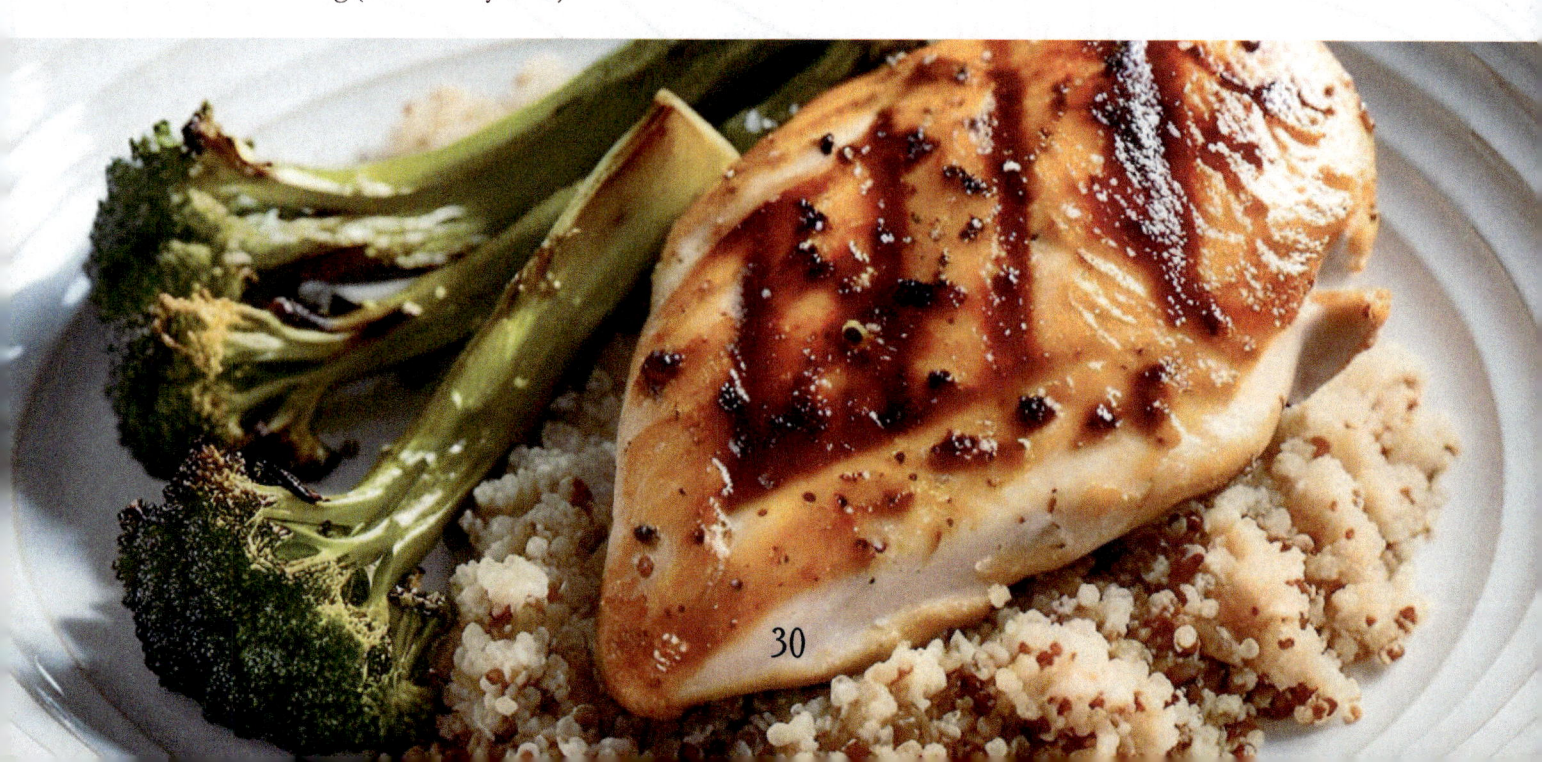

Cauliflower Rice Stir-Fry with Tofu and Veggies

- Prep Time: 10 minutes
- Cook Time: 15 minutes
- Total Time: 25 minutes
- Servings: 2

INGREDIENTS :

- 2 cups cauliflower rice (store-bought or homemade)
- 1 tbsp sesame oil (or olive oil)
- 1/2 cup tofu, cubed
- 1/2 cup bell peppers, chopped
- 1/2 cup carrots, shredded
- 1/4 cup peas (frozen or fresh)
- 2 tbsp soy sauce (low-sodium)
- 1 tsp grated ginger
- 1/4 cup green onions, sliced (optional)
- 1 tbsp sesame seeds (optional)

NUTRITIONAL BREAKDOWN (PER SERVING):

- Calories: 320
- Carbs: 20g (7% of daily value)
- Protein: 18g (36% of daily value)
- Fiber: 8g (32% of daily value)
- Fats: 22g (34% of daily value)

HOW TO MAKE :

1. Heat sesame oil in a large skillet over medium heat. Add the tofu cubes and cook until golden brown on all sides (about 5-7 minutes). Remove the tofu and set aside.
2. In the same skillet, add bell peppers, carrots, and peas. Stir-fry for 3-4 minutes until the veggies are tender-crisp
3. Add cauliflower rice to the skillet and cook for another 3-5 minutes, stirring occasionally.
4. Stir in soy sauce, ginger, and cooked tofu. Cook for 1-2 more minutes, allowing the flavors to combine.
5. Garnish with green onions and sesame seeds, and serve immediately.

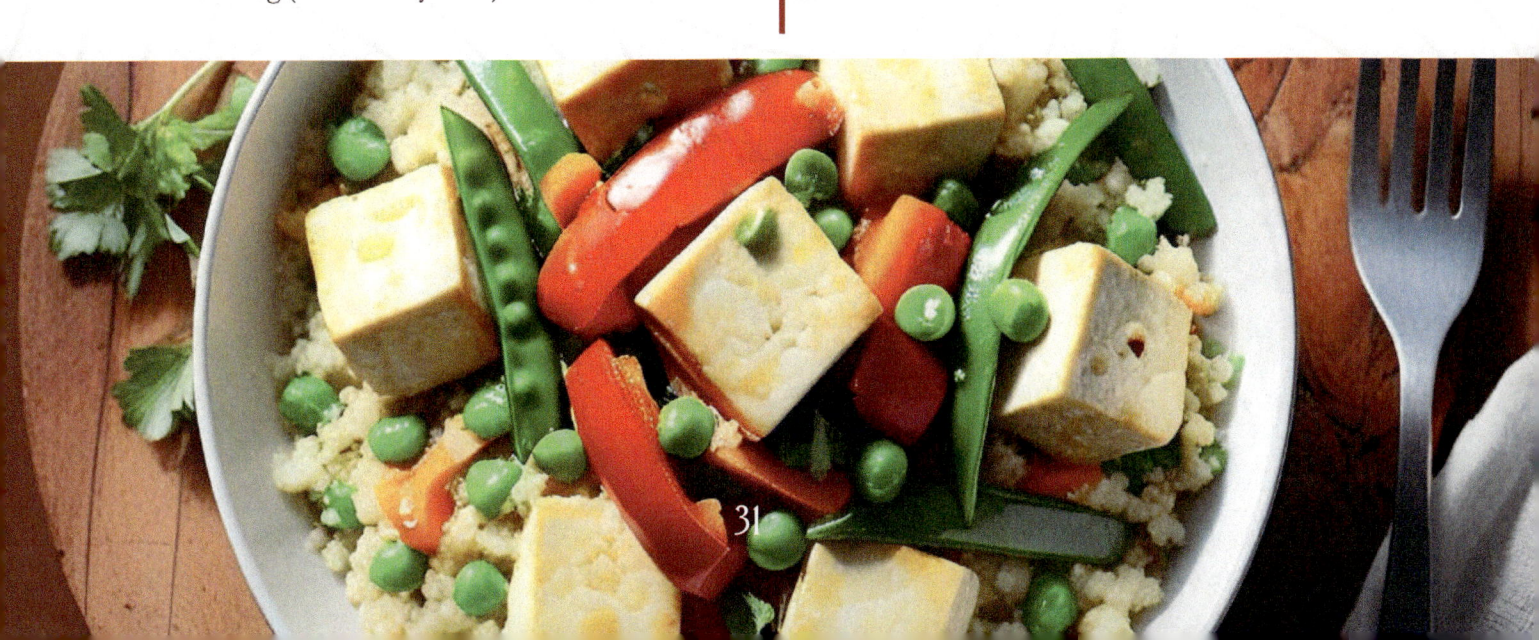

Spaghetti Squash with Ground Turkey and Marinara Sauce

- Prep Time: 10 minutes
- Cook Time: 30 minutes
- Total Time: 40 minutes
- Servings: 2

INGREDIENTS :

- 1 medium spaghetti squash
- 1 tbsp olive oil
- 1/2 lb ground turkey (lean)
- 1 cup marinara sauce (low-sodium, no added sugar)
- 1/4 cup Parmesan cheese, grated (optional)
- 1/4 tsp red pepper flakes (optional)
- Salt and pepper, to taste
- Fresh basil, for garnish (optional)

NUTRITIONAL BREAKDOWN (PER SERVING):

- Calories: 350
- Carbs: 20g (7% of daily value)
- Protein: 28g (56% of daily value)
- Fiber: 8g (32% of daily value)
- Fats: 18g (28% of daily value)

HOW TO MAKE :

1. Preheat the oven to 400°F (200°C). Cut the spaghetti squash in half lengthwise and remove the seeds. Drizzle with olive oil, salt, and pepper, then roast, cut side down, on a baking sheet for 30 minutes, or until tender.
2. While the squash roasts, heat olive oil in a pan over medium heat. Add ground turkey and cook until browned and fully cooked (about 5-7 minutes). Add marinara sauce to the turkey, stir to combine, and simmer for 5 minutes.
3. Once the squash is roasted, use a fork to scrape the flesh into spaghetti-like strands.
4. Top the spaghetti squash with the turkey marinara sauce, grated Parmesan, and a sprinkle of red pepper flakes, if desired. Garnish with fresh basil.

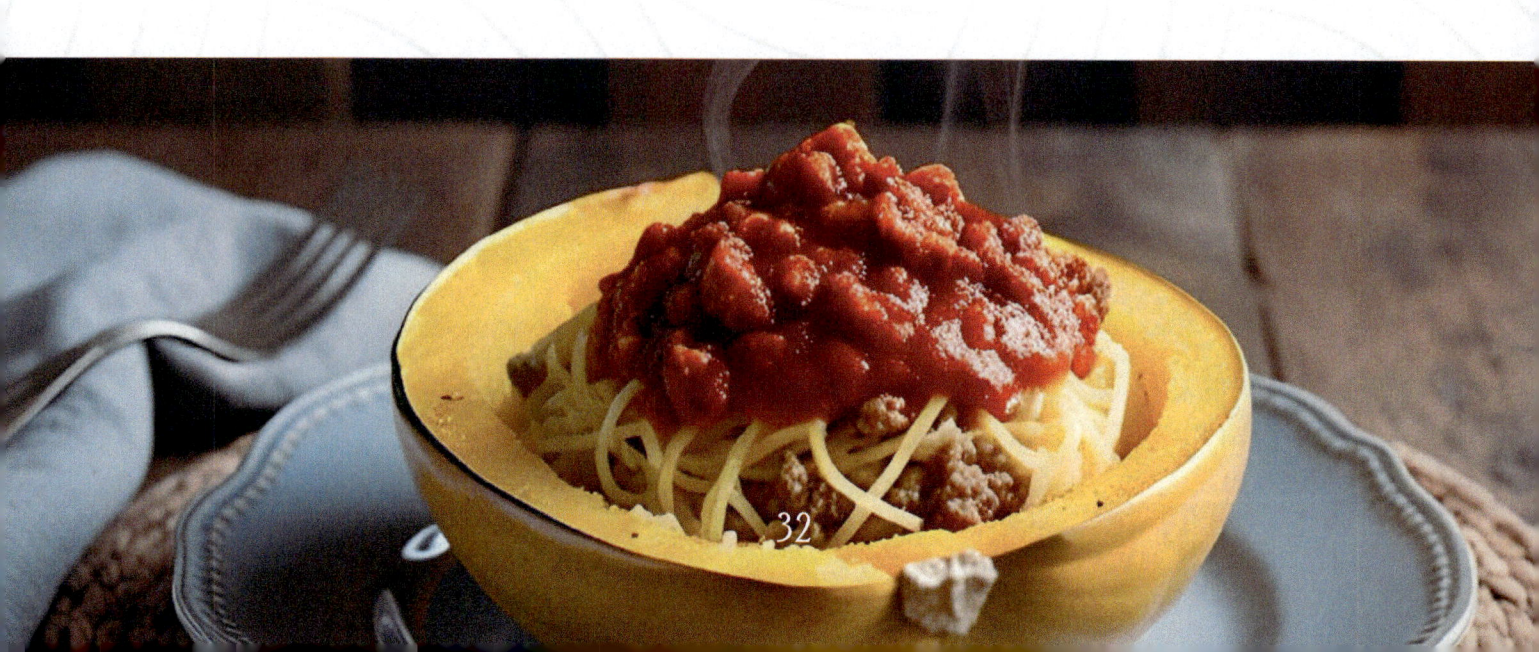

Baked Cod with Lemon and Asparagus

- Prep Time: 5 minutes
- Cook Time: 20 minutes
- Total Time: 25 minutes
- Servings: 2

INGREDIENTS :

- 2 cod fillets (4 oz each)
- 1 tbsp olive oil
- 1 tsp lemon zest
- 1 tbsp fresh lemon juice
- Salt and pepper, to taste
- 1 bunch asparagus, trimmed
- 1 tsp garlic powder
- 1 tbsp fresh parsley, chopped (optional)

NUTRITIONAL BREAKDOWN (PER SERVING):

- Calories: 320
- Carbs: 12g (4% of daily value)
- Protein: 32g (64% of daily value)
- Fiber: 6g (24% of daily value)
- Fats: 18g (28% of daily value)

HOW TO MAKE :

1. Preheat the oven to 400°F (200°C). Place the cod fillets on a baking sheet lined with parchment paper. Drizzle with olive oil, lemon zest, lemon juice, salt, and pepper.
2. Arrange the asparagus around the fish on the baking sheet. Sprinkle it with garlic powder and season with salt and pepper.
3. Roast for 15-20 minutes, or until the cod is cooked through and flakes easily with a fork.
4. Garnish with fresh parsley and serve with the roasted asparagus.

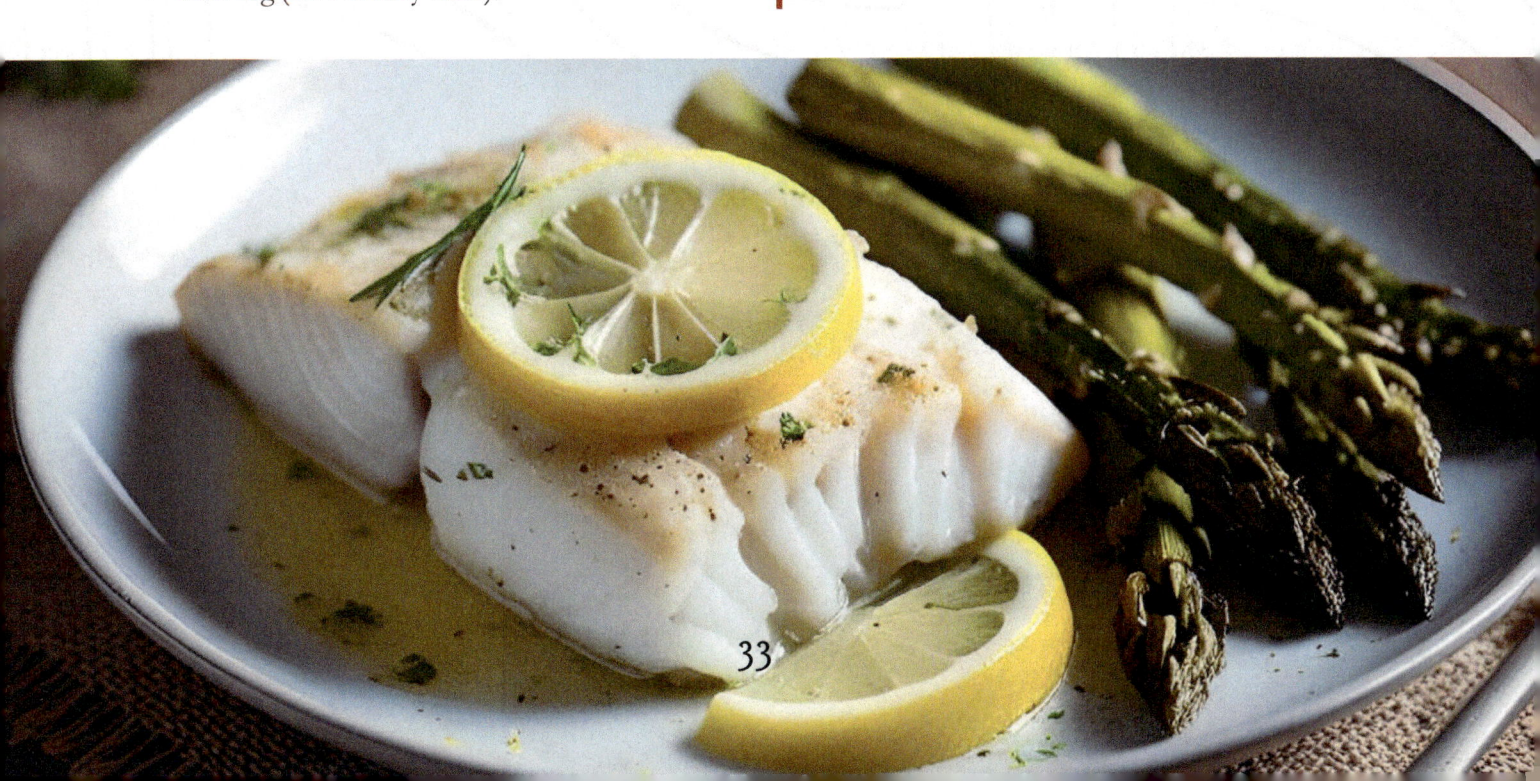

Turkey Meatballs with Zucchini Noodles

- Prep Time: 10 minutes
- Cook Time: 25 minutes
- Total Time: 35 minutes
- Servings: 2

INGREDIENTS :

- 1 lb ground turkey (lean)
- 1/4 cup almond flour (or breadcrumbs)
- 1 egg
- 1 tbsp Italian seasoning
- 1/2 tsp garlic powder
- Salt and pepper, to taste
- 2 medium zucchinis, spiralized into noodles
- 1 cup marinara sauce (low-sodium, no added sugar)
- 1 tbsp olive oil

NUTRITIONAL BREAKDOWN (PER SERVING):

- Calories: 400
- Carbs: 20g (7% of daily value)
- Protein: 35g (70% of daily value)
- Fiber: 6g (24% of daily value)
- Fats: 22g (34% of daily value)

HOW TO MAKE :

1. Preheat the oven to 375°F (190°C). In a bowl, combine the ground turkey, almond flour, egg, Italian seasoning, garlic powder, salt, and pepper. Mix well and form into 12 small meatballs.
2. Place the meatballs on a baking sheet lined with parchment paper. Bake for 20-25 minutes, or until cooked through and golden brown
3. While the meatballs cook, heat olive oil in a skillet over medium heat. Add zucchini noodles and sauté for 2-3 minutes until just tender.
4. Warm the marinara sauce in a small pot. Serve the meatballs on top of the zucchini noodles and drizzle with marinara sauce.

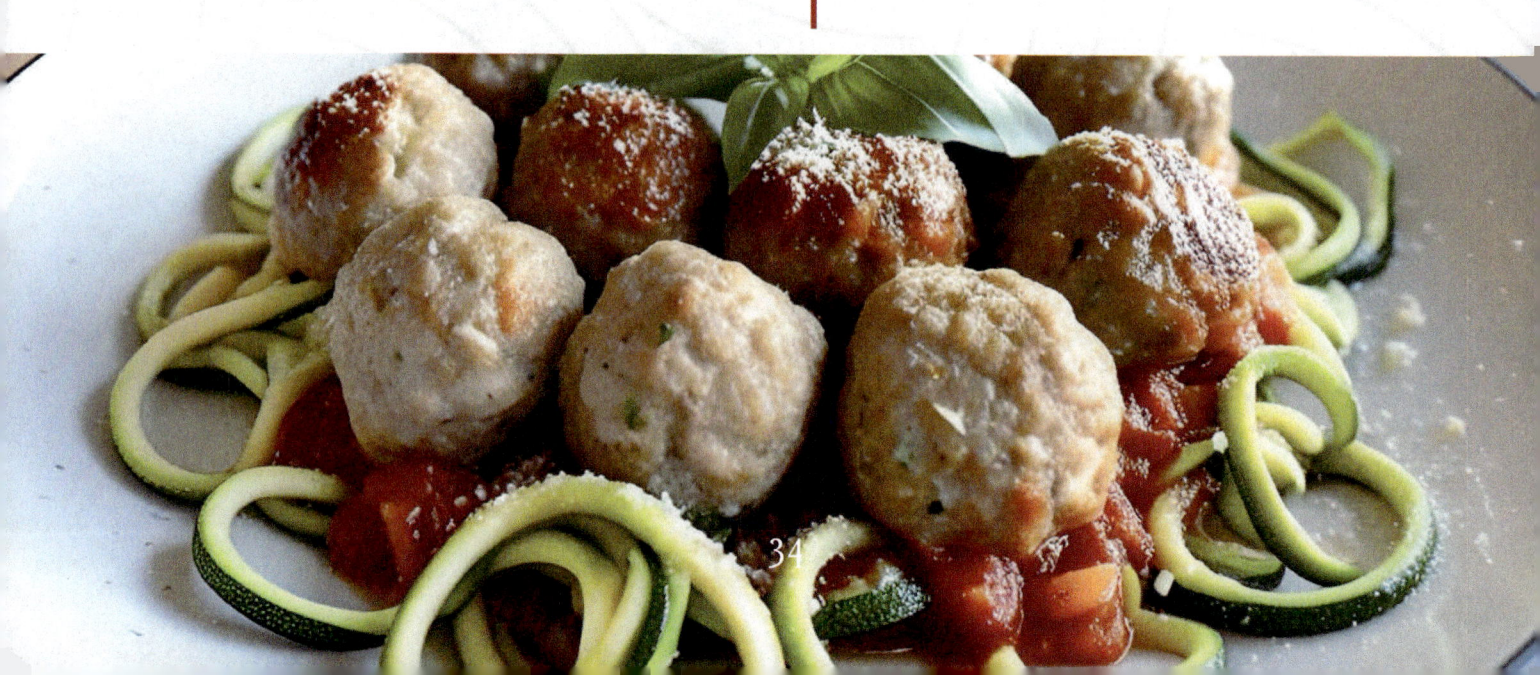

Stir-Fried Shrimp with Bell Peppers and Brown Rice

- Prep Time: 10 minutes
- Cook Time: 15 minutes
- Total Time: 25 minutes
- Servings: 2

INGREDIENTS :

- 1 lb shrimp, peeled and deveined
- 1 tbsp olive oil
- 1 bell pepper, thinly sliced
- 1 small onion, thinly sliced
- 1 cup cooked brown rice
- 2 cloves garlic, minced
- 1 tbsp soy sauce (low-sodium)
- 1 tsp sesame oil (optional)
- 1 tbsp sesame seeds (optional)
- Salt and pepper, to taste

NUTRITIONAL BREAKDOWN (PER SERVING):

- Calories: 350
- Carbs: 38g (13% of daily value)
- Protein: 28g (56% of daily value)
- Fiber: 5g (20% of daily value)
- Fats: 12g (18% of daily value)

HOW TO MAKE :

1. Heat olive oil in a large skillet over medium-high heat. Add the shrimp and cook for 2-3 minutes per side until pink and opaque. Remove the shrimp from the skillet and set aside.
2. In the same skillet, add the bell pepper, onion, and garlic. Stir-fry for 3-4 minutes, until the vegetables are tender.
3. Add the cooked brown rice to the skillet and stir to combine with the vegetables. Drizzle with soy sauce and sesame oil, if using. Add the shrimp back into the skillet and stir to combine. Cook for an additional 2 minutes, just until everything is heated through.
4. Garnish with sesame seeds, if desired, and serve immediately.

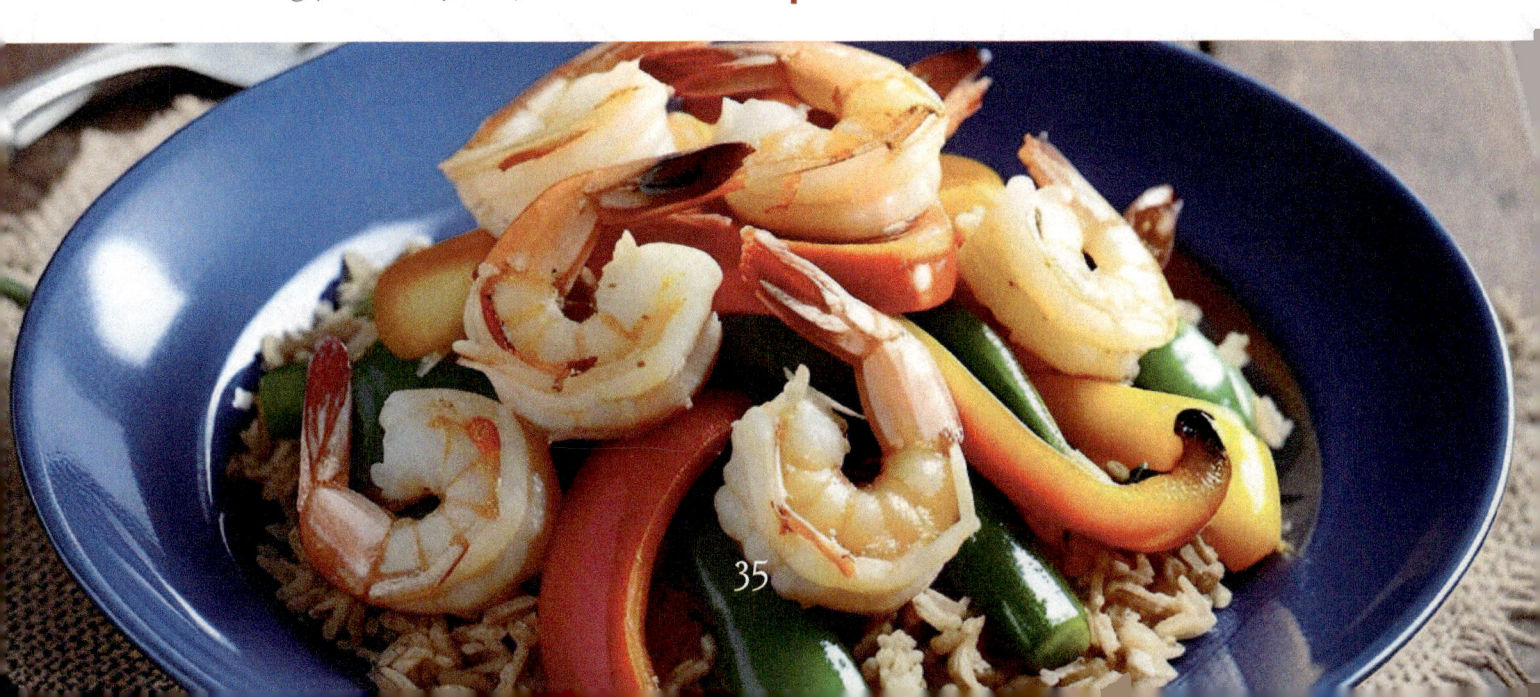

Roasted Chicken with Brussels Sprouts and Sweet Potato

- Prep Time: 10 minutes
- Cook Time: 35 minutes
- Total Time: 45 minutes
- Servings: 2

INGREDIENTS :

- 2 bone-in, skin-on chicken thighs
- 1 tbsp olive oil
- 1/2 tsp paprika
- 1/2 tsp garlic powder
- Salt and pepper, to taste
- 1 cup Brussels sprouts, halved
- 1 medium sweet potato, diced
- 1 tbsp fresh thyme (optional)

NUTRITIONAL BREAKDOWN (PER SERVING):

- Calories: 450
- Carbs: 35g (12% of daily value)
- Protein: 35g (70% of daily value)
- Fiber: 9g (36% of daily value)
- Fats: 22g (34% of daily value)

HOW TO MAKE :

1. Preheat your oven to 400°F (200°C). Rub the chicken thighs with olive oil, paprika, garlic powder, salt, and pepper.
2. On a baking sheet, arrange the chicken thighs, Brussels sprouts, and sweet potato. Drizzle everything with a little more olive oil and season with salt and pepper.
3. Roast in the oven for 35 minutes, or until the chicken reaches an internal temperature of 165°F (75°C) and the vegetables are tender.
4. Garnish with fresh thyme, if desired, and serve immediately.

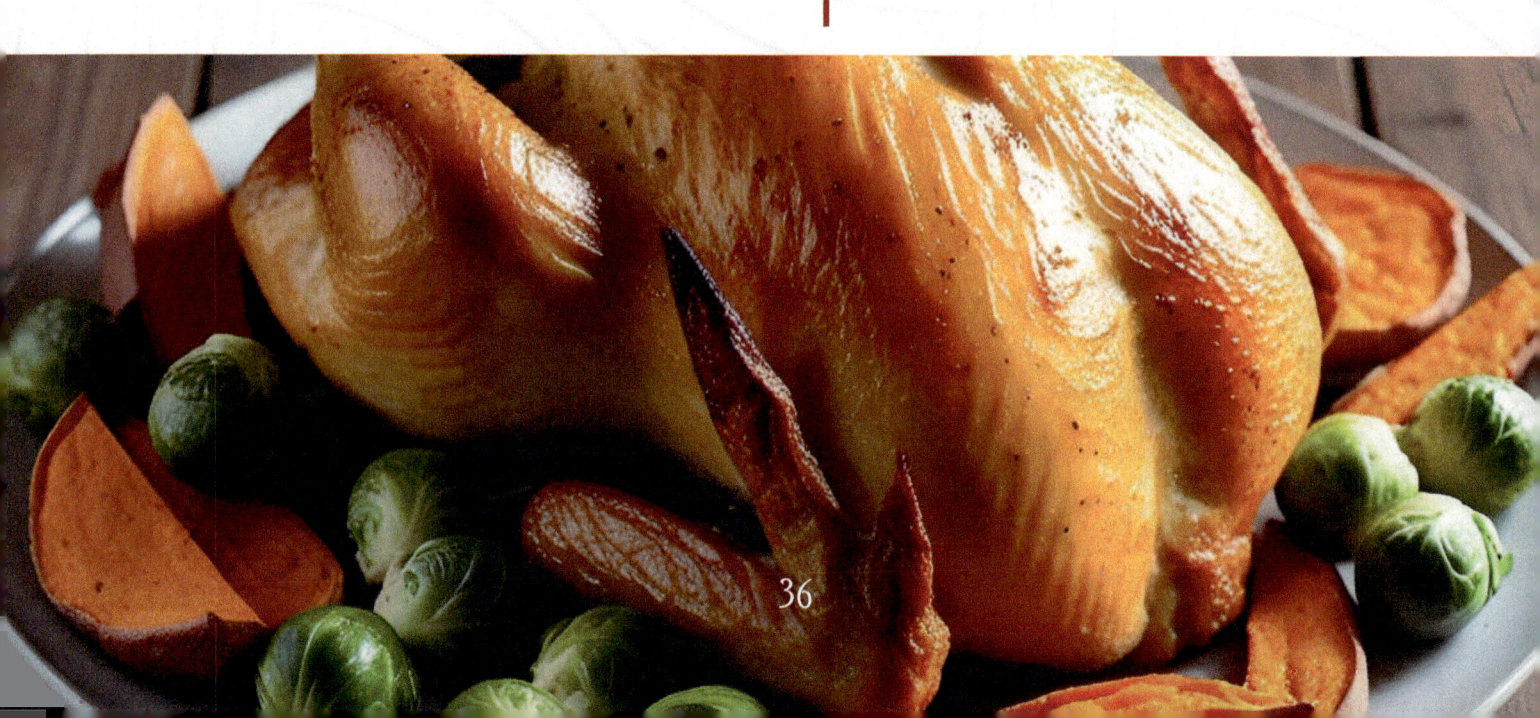

Stuffed Bell Peppers with Quinoa and Ground Beef

- Prep Time: 15 minutes
- Cook Time: 30 minutes
- Total Time: 45 minutes
- Servings: 2

INGREDIENTS :

- 2 large bell peppers, tops cut off and seeds removed
- 1/2 lb ground beef (lean)
- 1/2 cup cooked quinoa
- 1/4 cup onion, chopped
- 1/4 cup diced tomatoes
- 1 tbsp olive oil
- 1 tsp cumin
- Salt and pepper, to taste
- 1/4 cup shredded cheese (optional, for topping)

NUTRITIONAL BREAKDOWN (PER SERVING):

- Calories: 380
- Carbs: 25g (8% of daily value)
- Protein: 30g (60% of daily value)
- Fiber: 8g (32% of daily value)
- Fats: 20g (31% of daily value)

HOW TO MAKE :

1. Preheat your oven to 375°F (190°C). Place the bell peppers on a baking sheet.
2. Heat olive oil in a skillet over medium heat. Add ground beef and cook, breaking it apart, until browned. Add onion and cook for an additional 3-4 minutes.
3. Stir in quinoa, diced tomatoes, cumin, salt, and pepper. Mix until everything is well combined.
4. Stuff the bell peppers with the beef and quinoa mixture and place them on the baking sheet.
5. Cover with aluminum foil and bake for 25 minutes. If using cheese, sprinkle it on top of the peppers during the last 5 minutes of baking, and cook until melted and bubbly.
6. Serve hot and enjoy!

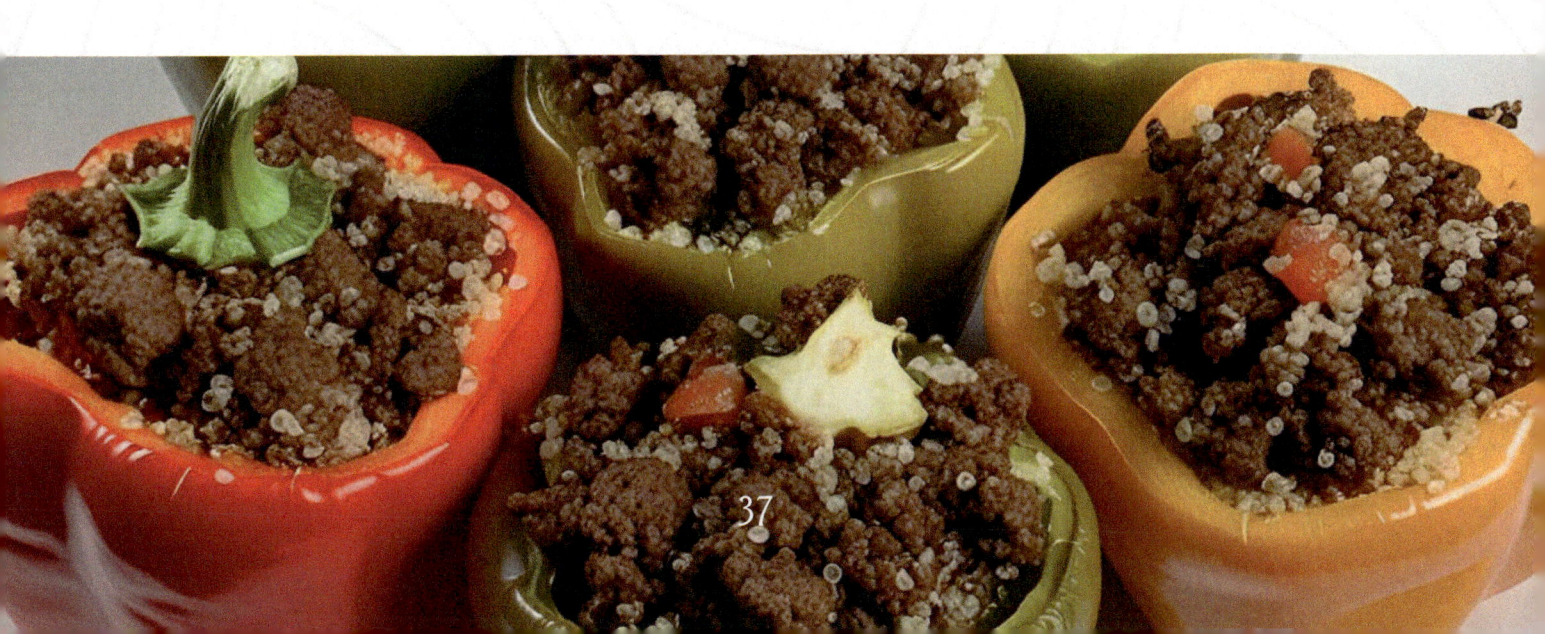

Chapter 5: Vegetarian Recipes (Plant-Based Power for Balanced Blood Sugar)

When managing prediabetes, embracing plant-based meals is a game-changer. Plant-based foods are naturally high in fiber, low in fat, and rich in antioxidants all key components that help stabilize blood sugar levels. These meals are not only good for you but also for your heart, your digestive system, and your overall well-being. Plus, they're delicious, satisfying, and easy to prepare, with ingredients that are readily available at your local grocery store.

Chickpea and Spinach Stew

- Prep Time: 10 minutes
- Cook Time: 20 minutes
- Total Time: 30 minutes
- Servings: 2

INGREDIENTS :

- 1 can (15 oz) chickpeas, drained and rinsed
- 1 tbsp olive oil
- 1 onion, chopped
- 2 cloves garlic, minced
- 2 cups spinach (fresh or frozen)
- 1 can (14 oz) diced tomatoes
- 1/2 tsp cumin
- 1/2 tsp turmeric
- 1/4 tsp paprika
- Salt and pepper, to taste
- 1 tbsp lemon juice (optional)

NUTRITIONAL BREAKDOWN (PER SERVING):

- Calories: 300
- Carbs: 45g (15% of daily value)
- Protein: 15g (30% of daily value)
- Fiber: 12g (48% of daily value)
- Fats: 12g (18% of daily value)

HOW TO MAKE :

1. Heat olive oil in a large pot over medium heat. Add the onion and garlic, cooking for about 5 minutes until softened.
2. Add the chickpeas, diced tomatoes, cumin, turmeric, paprika, salt, and pepper. Stir to combine.
3. Add the spinach and cook until wilted (about 2-3 minutes).
4. If using fresh spinach, you may need to add a bit of water or vegetable broth to achieve your desired consistency.
5. Simmer for another 5-7 minutes, allowing the flavors to meld together.
6. Squeeze in some fresh lemon juice before serving for a touch of brightness.

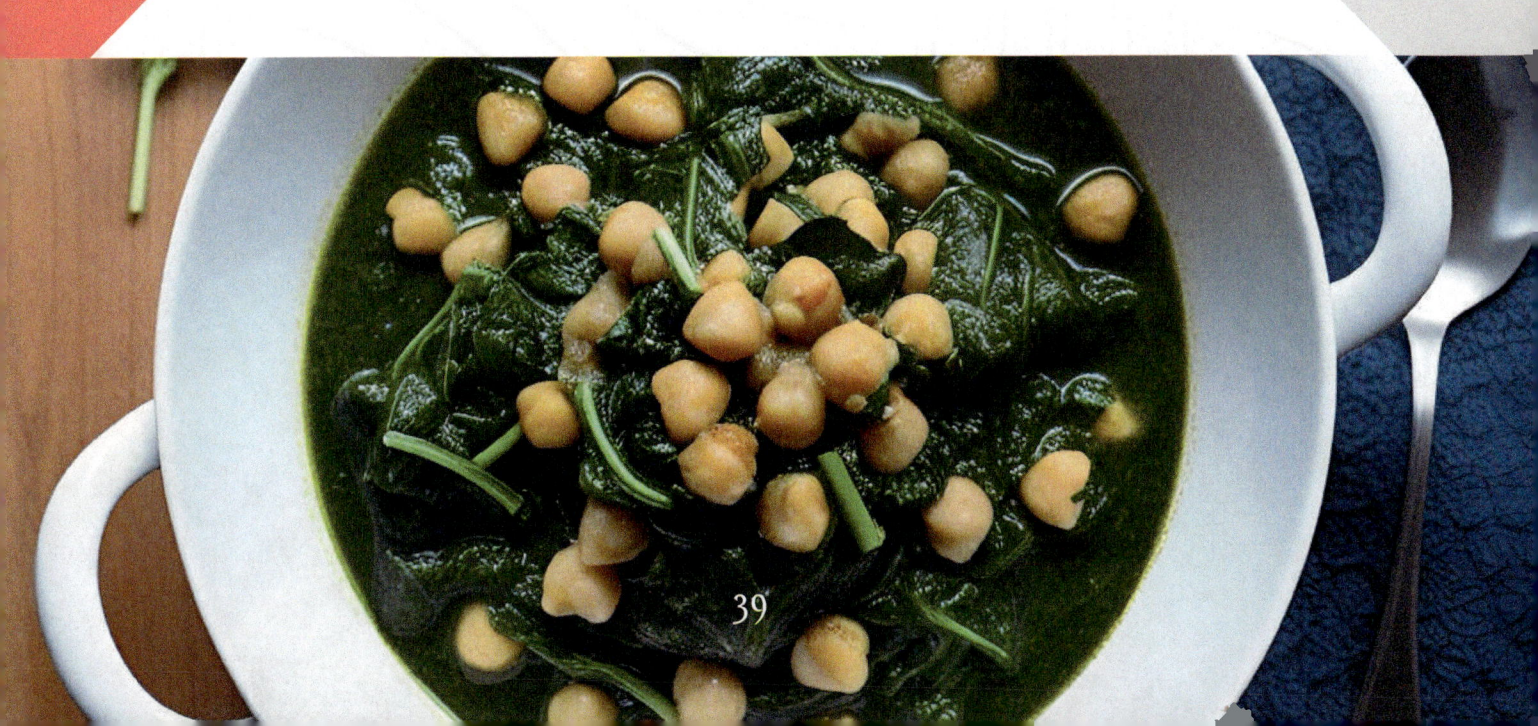

Lentil Tacos with Avocado and Salsa

- Prep Time: 10 minutes
- Cook Time: 15 minutes
- Total Time: 25 minutes
- Servings: 2

INGREDIENTS :

- 1 cup cooked lentils (or 1 can lentils, drained and rinsed)
- 1 tbsp olive oil
- 1 tsp chili powder
- 1/2 tsp cumin
- 1/2 tsp garlic powder
- Salt and pepper, to taste
- 4 small corn tortillas
- 1/2 avocado, sliced
- 1/4 cup salsa
- Fresh cilantro, for garnish

NUTRITIONAL BREAKDOWN (PER SERVING):

- Calories: 320
- Carbs: 45g (15% of daily value)
- Protein: 15g (30% of daily value)
- Fiber: 14g (56% of daily value)
- Fats: 12g (18% of daily value)

HOW TO MAKE :

1. Heat olive oil in a skillet over medium heat. Add the cooked lentils, chili powder, cumin, garlic powder, salt, and pepper. Stir to coat the lentils evenly with the spices.
2. Cook for 5-7 minutes, stirring occasionally, until the lentils are heated through and slightly crispy on the edges.
3. Warm the corn tortillas in a dry skillet or microwave for 30 seconds.
4. To assemble the tacos, spoon the seasoned lentils onto each tortilla and top with sliced avocado, salsa, and a sprinkle of fresh cilantro.
5. Serve immediately and enjoy!

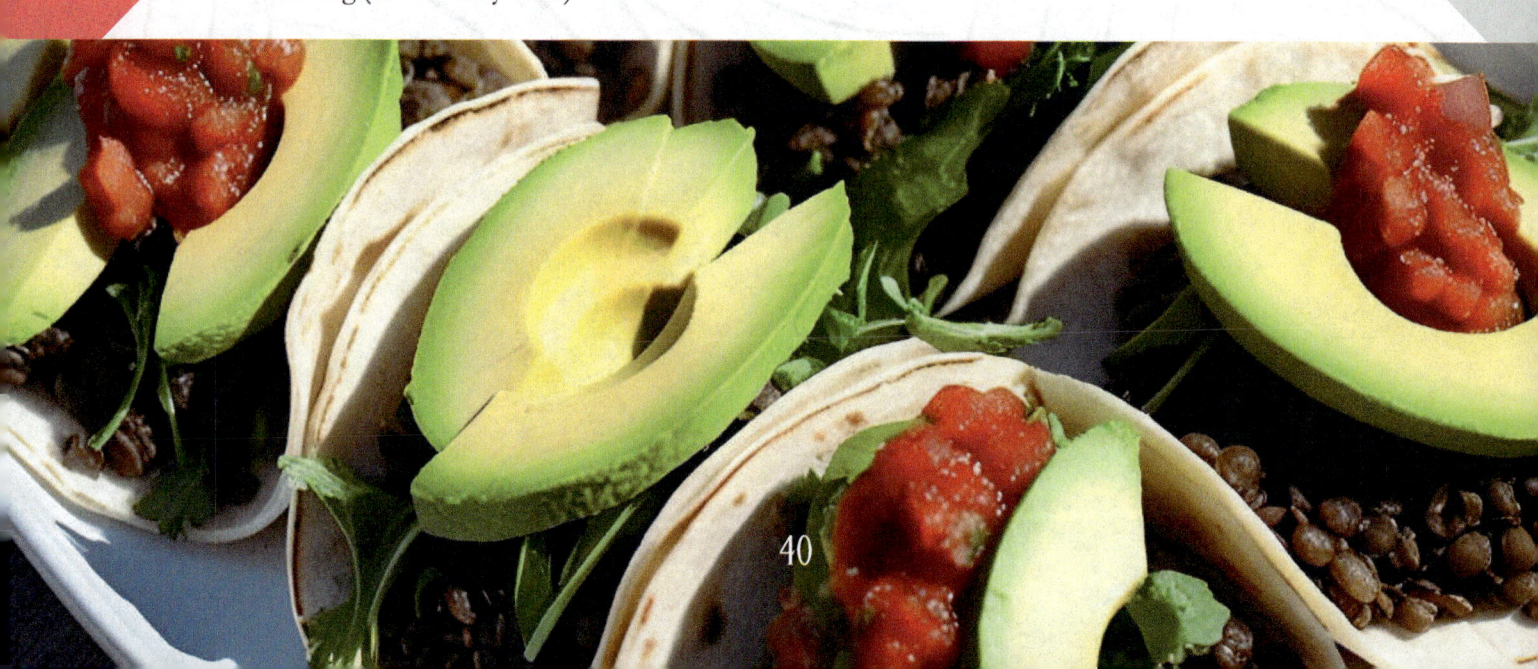

Stuffed Sweet Potatoes with Black Beans and Quinoa

- Prep Time: 10 minutes
- Cook Time: 30 minutes
- Total Time: 40 minutes
- Servings: 2

INGREDIENTS :

- 2 medium sweet potatoes
- 1/2 cup cooked quinoa
- 1 can (15 oz) black beans, drained and rinsed
- 1/4 cup red onion, diced
- 1/4 cup cilantro, chopped
- 1 tbsp lime juice
- 1 tsp cumin
- Salt and pepper, to taste
- /4 cup plain Greek yogurt (optional, for topping)

NUTRITIONAL BREAKDOWN (PER SERVING):

- Calories: 400
- Carbs: 65g (22% of daily value)
- Protein: 14g (28% of daily value)
- Fiber: 12g (48% of daily value)
- Fats: 10g (15% of daily value)

HOW TO MAKE :

1. Preheat your oven to 400°F (200°C). Pierce the sweet potatoes a few times with a fork and place them on a baking sheet. Roast for 30 minutes, or until tender.
2. While the sweet potatoes are roasting, cook the quinoa according to package instructions.
3. In a bowl, mix the black beans, red onion, cilantro, lime juice, cumin, salt, and pepper.
4. Once the sweet potatoes are roasted and tender, cut them open and fluff the insides with a fork.
5. Top each sweet potato with the black bean and quinoa mixture. Optionally, add a dollop of Greek yogurt for a creamy texture.
6. Serve immediately.

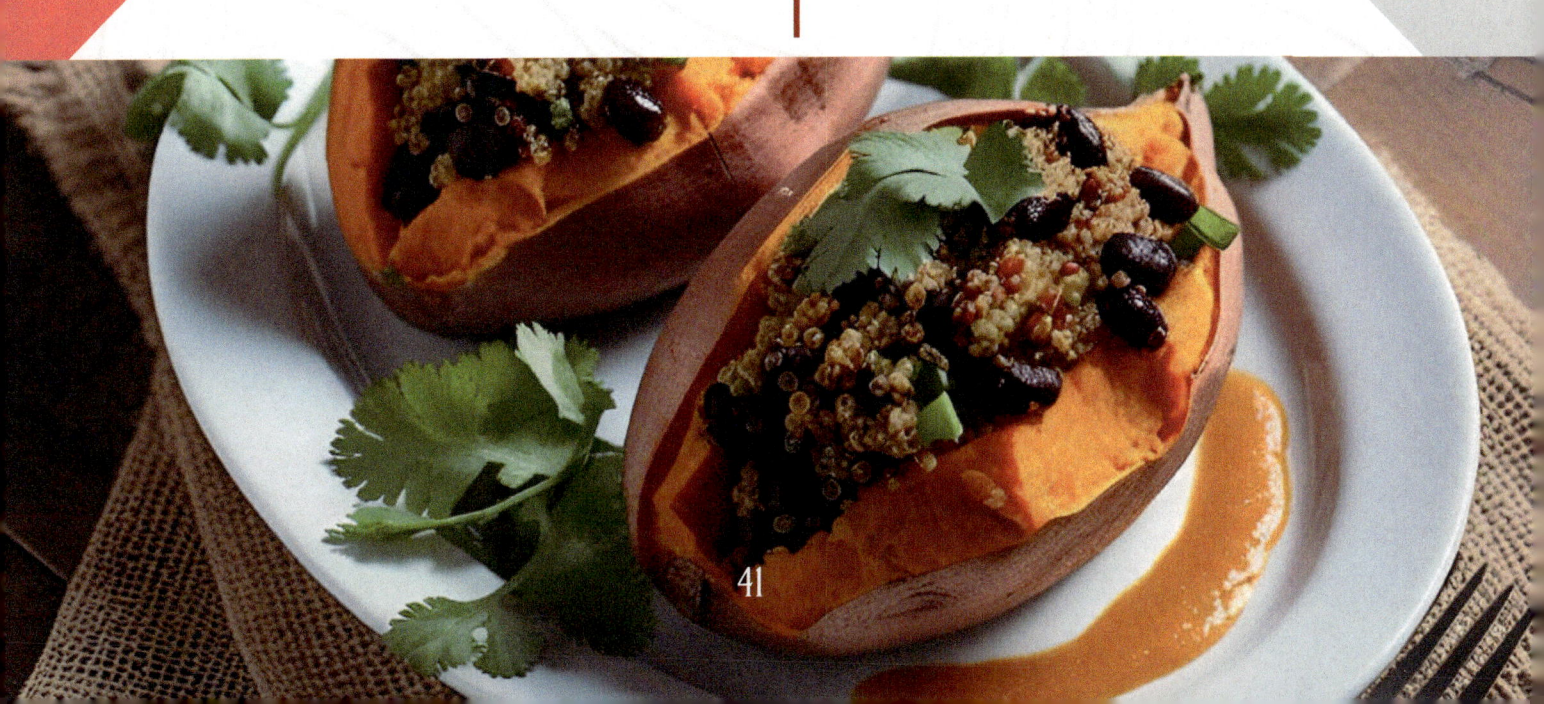

Cauliflower Rice Stir-Fry with Tofu and Vegetables

- Prep Time: 10 minutes
- Cook Time: 15 minutes
- Total Time: 25 minutes
- Servings: 2

INGREDIENTS :

- 2 cups cauliflower rice (store-bought or homemade)
- 1 tbsp sesame oil (or olive oil)
- 1/2 block firm tofu, cubed
- 1/2 cup bell peppers, diced
- 1/2 cup carrots, shredded
- 1/4 cup peas (frozen or fresh)
- 2 tbsp soy sauce (low-sodium)
- 1 tsp grated ginger
- 1/4 cup green onions, sliced (optional)
- 1 tbsp sesame seeds (optional)

NUTRITIONAL BREAKDOWN (PER SERVING):

- Calories: 250
- Carbs: 20g (7% of daily value)
- Protein: 12g (24% of daily value)
- Fiber: 8g (32% of daily value)
- Fats: 16g (24% of daily value)

HOW TO MAKE :

1. Heat sesame oil in a large skillet over medium heat. Add the tofu cubes and cook for 5-7 minutes, or until golden brown and crispy.
2. Add the bell peppers, carrots, and peas to the skillet and stir-fry for 3-4 minutes until the vegetables are tender-crisp.
3. Add the cauliflower rice and cook for another 3-5 minutes, stirring occasionally.
4. Stir in soy sauce, ginger, and green onions. Cook for an additional 2 minutes, allowing the flavors to meld together.
5. Garnish with sesame seeds (if desired) and serve immediately.

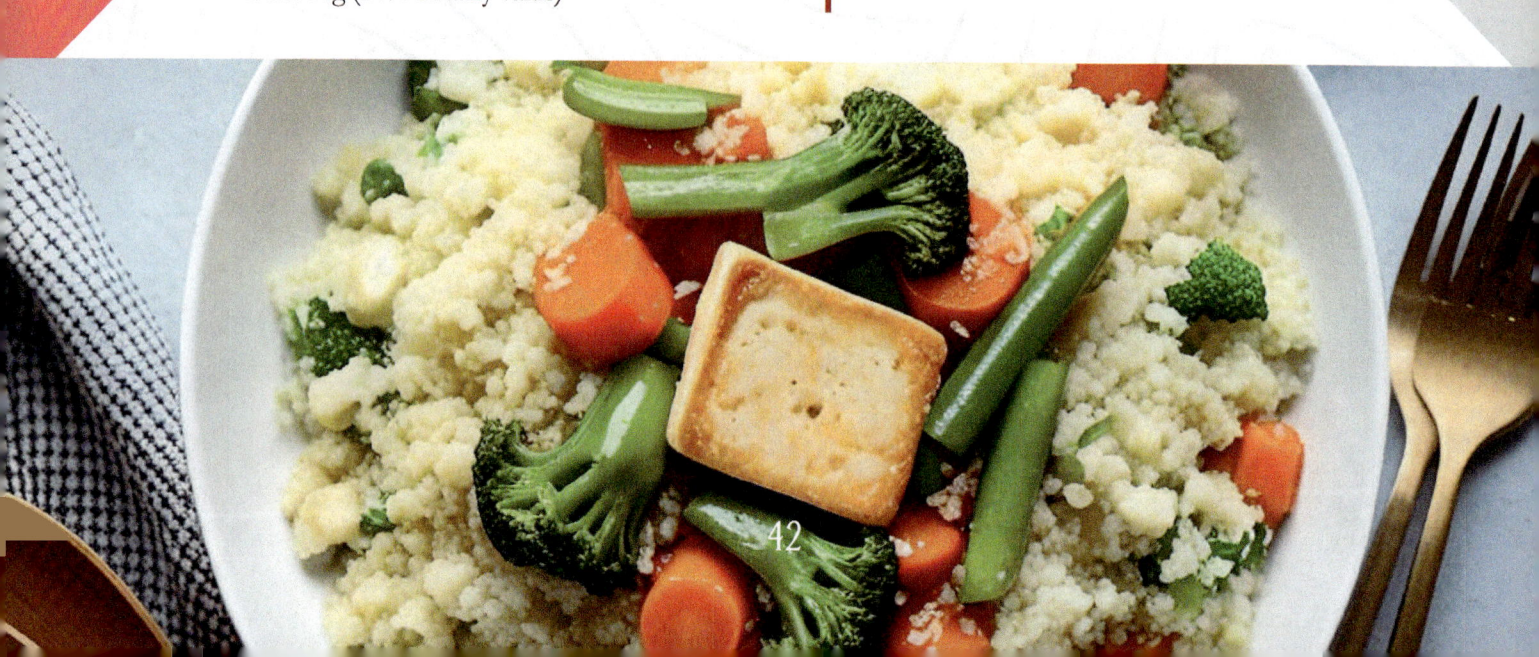

Zucchini and Mushroom Risotto

- Prep Time: 10 minutes
- Cook Time: 20 minutes
- Total Time: 30 minutes
- Servings: 2

INGREDIENTS :

- 1 tbsp olive oil
- 1 small onion, finely chopped
- 2 medium zucchinis, diced
- 1 cup mushrooms, sliced
- 1 cup Arborio rice (risotto rice)
- 2 cups vegetable broth (low-sodium)
- 1/4 cup dry white wine (optional)
- 1/2 cup Parmesan cheese (optional)
- 1/4 cup fresh parsley, chopped
- Salt and pepper, to taste

NUTRITIONAL BREAKDOWN (PER SERVING):

- Calories: 350
- Carbs: 50g (17% of daily value)
- Protein: 8g (16% of daily value)
- Fiber: 6g (24% of daily value)
- Fats: 14g (22% of daily value)

HOW TO MAKE :

1. Heat olive oil in a large skillet over medium heat. Add the onion and cook for about 3-4 minutes, until soft.
2. Add the zucchini and mushrooms, cooking for another 5-7 minutes until tender.
3. Stir in the Arborio rice, coating it with the vegetables and oil.
4. If using, pour in the white wine and cook until it evaporates.
5. Gradually add vegetable broth, 1/2 cup at a time, stirring constantly and letting the rice absorb the liquid before adding more.
6. Continue until the rice is cooked through and creamy (about 18-20 minutes).
7. Stir in Parmesan (if using), fresh parsley, and season with salt and pepper.
8. Serve immediately, garnished with additional parsley.

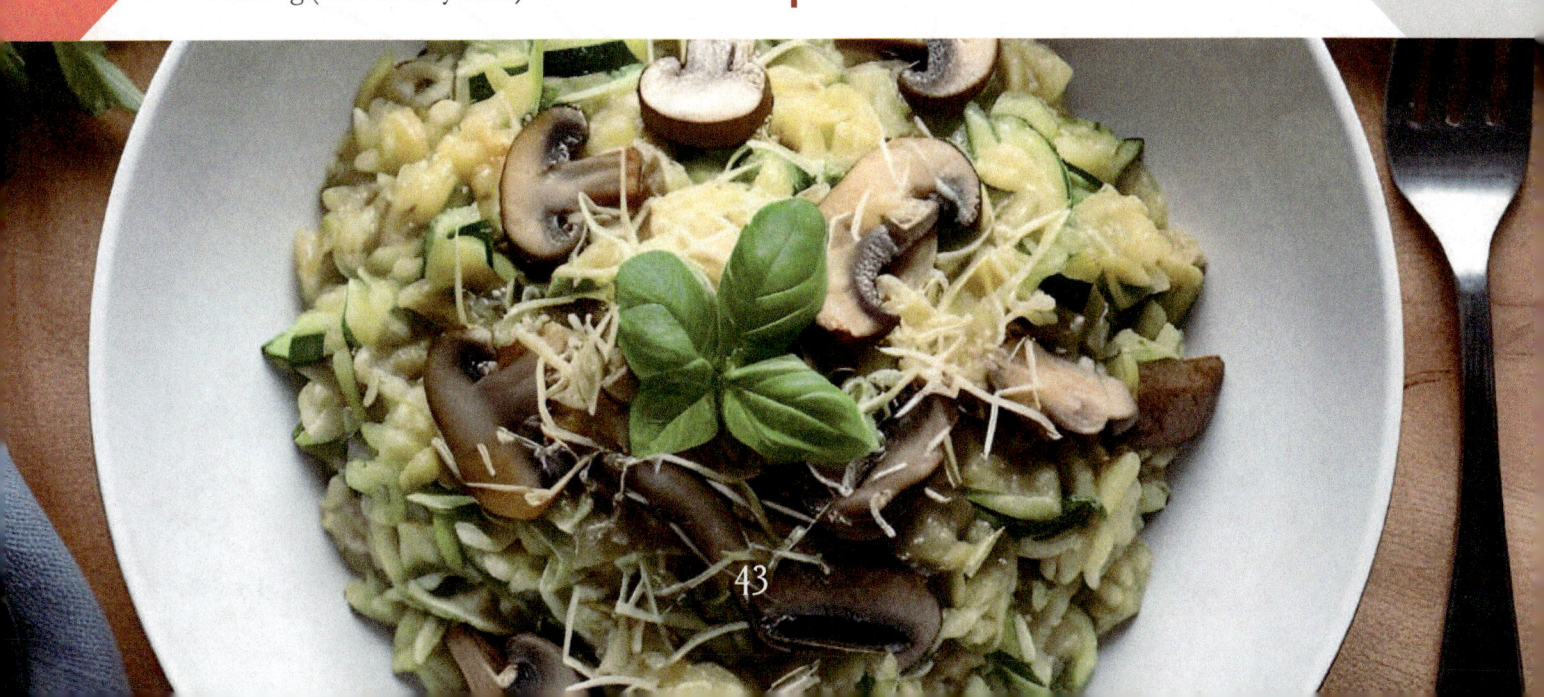

Eggplant Parmesan with a Low-Glycemic Tomato Sauce

- Prep Time: 15 minutes
- Cook Time: 30 minutes
- Total Time: 45 minutes
- Servings: 2

INGREDIENTS :

- 1 medium eggplant, sliced into rounds
- 1 cup almond flour (for breading)
- 1/2 cup egg whites (or 1 egg)
- 2 cups low-glycemic tomato sauce (preferably homemade or no-sugar-added)
- 1/4 cup fresh basil, chopped
- 1/4 cup mozzarella cheese (optional)
- 1 tbsp olive oil
- Salt and pepper, to taste

NUTRITIONAL BREAKDOWN (PER SERVING):

- Calories: 280
- Carbs: 18g (6% of daily value)
- Protein: 12g (24% of daily value)
- Fiber: 8g (32% of daily value)
- Fats: 18g (28% of daily value)

HOW TO MAKE :

1. Preheat your oven to 375°F (190°C). Lightly grease a baking sheet with olive oil.
2. Dip the eggplant slices into egg whites and then coat them with almond flour, ensuring they are evenly coated.
3. Arrange the breaded eggplant slices on the baking sheet and bake for 15-20 minutes, flipping halfway through, until golden and crispy.
4. While the eggplant is baking, warm the tomato sauce in a saucepan over medium heat.
5. Once the eggplant is baked, layer it in a baking dish, spooning tomato sauce over each layer.
6. Sprinkle with mozzarella cheese (optional) and bake for an additional 10 minutes, until the cheese is melted and bubbly.
7. Garnish with fresh basil before serving.

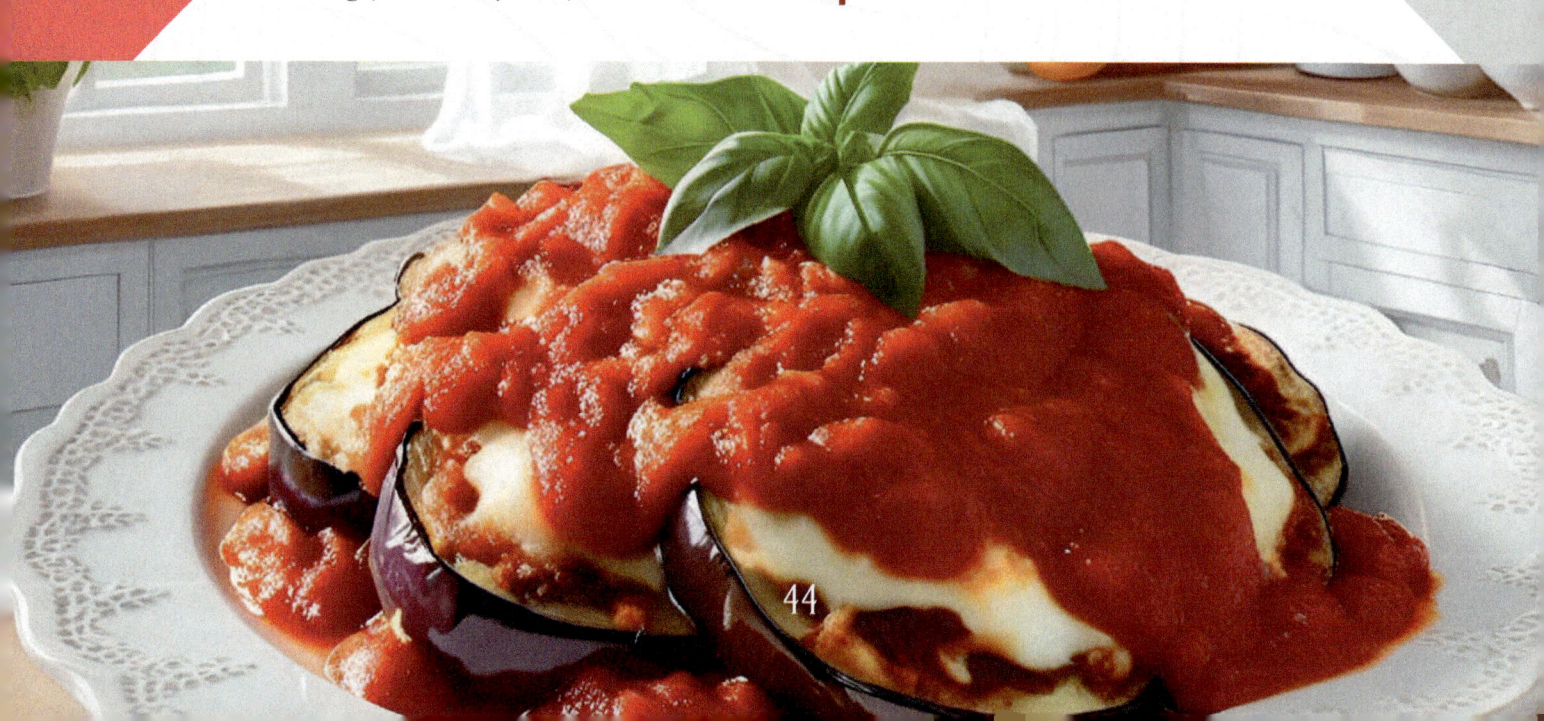

Spaghetti Squash with Pesto and Cherry Tomatoes

- Prep Time: 10 minutes
- Cook Time: 30 minutes
- Total Time: 40 minutes
- Servings: 2

INGREDIENTS :

- 1 medium spaghetti squash
- 1 tbsp olive oil
- 1 cup cherry tomatoes, halved
- 1/4 cup homemade or store-bought pesto (preferably low-sodium and without added sugars)
- 1 tbsp Parmesan cheese (optional)
- Salt and pepper, to taste

NUTRITIONAL BREAKDOWN (PER SERVING):

- Calories: 250
- Carbs: 20g (7% of daily value)
- Protein: 6g (12% of daily value)
- Fiber: 7g (28% of daily value)
- Fats: 18g (28% of daily value)

HOW TO MAKE :

1. Preheat the oven to 400°F (200°C). Cut the spaghetti squash in half lengthwise and scoop out the seeds
2. Drizzle the squash halves with olive oil and season with salt and pepper. Place them cut side down on a baking sheet and roast for 30 minutes, or until tender.
3. While the squash roasts, heat the pesto in a small saucepan over low heat. Add the cherry tomatoes and cook for 3-4 minutes, just until they soften.
4. Once the squash is roasted, use a fork to scrape out the flesh, creating "spaghetti-like" strands.
5. Toss the spaghetti squash with the pesto and cherry tomatoes, and sprinkle with Parmesan (if desired).
6. Serve immediately, garnished with extra basil or Parmesan.

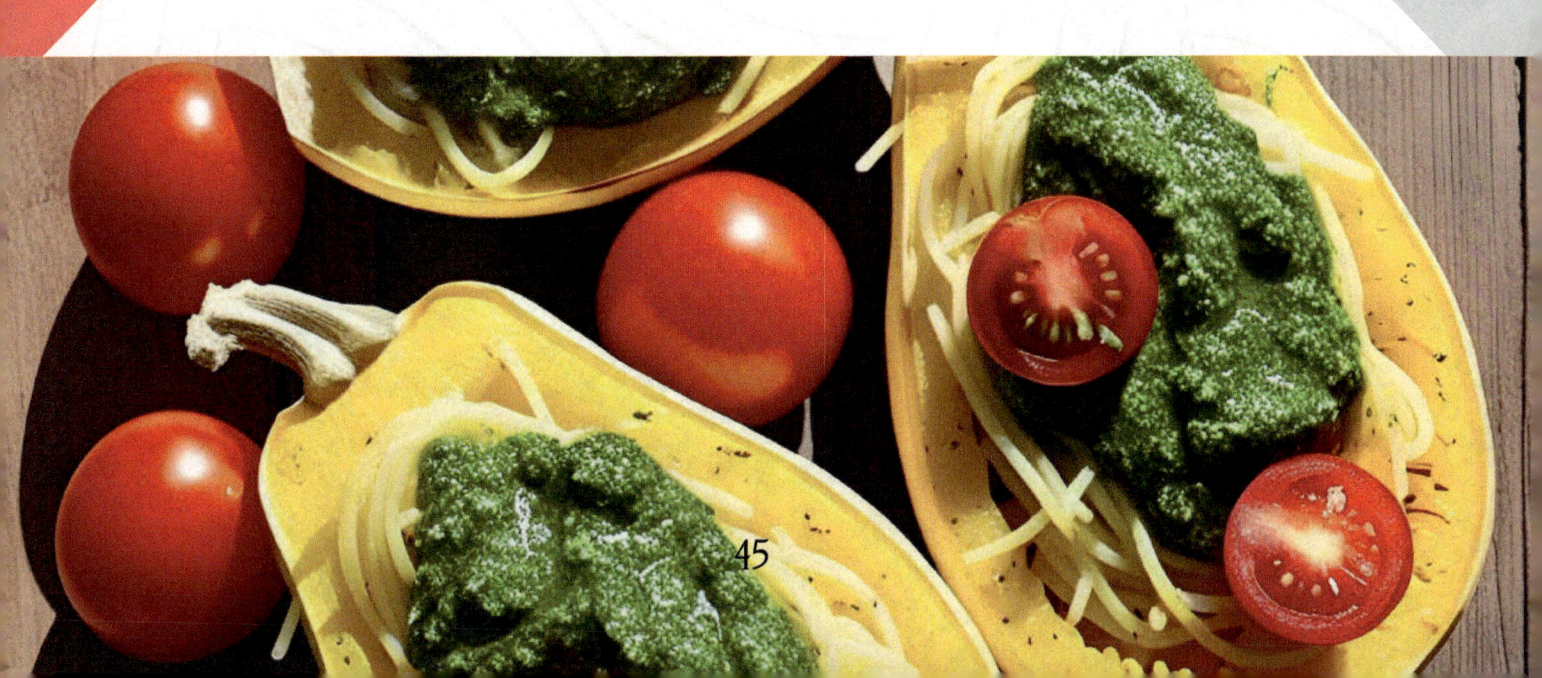

Lentil and Vegetable Curry with Brown Rice

- Prep Time: 10 minutes
- Cook Time: 35 minutes
- Total Time: 45 minutes
- Servings: 4

INGREDIENTS :

- 1 cup dry lentils, rinsed
- 1 tbsp olive oil
- 1 small onion, chopped
- 2 cloves garlic, minced
- 1 tbsp curry powder
- 1 can (14 oz) diced tomatoes
- 1/2 cup coconut milk (unsweetened)
- 1/2 cup carrots, chopped
- 1/2 cup cauliflower florets
- 1 cup spinach (fresh or frozen)
- 2 cups cooked brown rice
- Salt and pepper, to taste

HOW TO MAKE :

1. In a large pot, heat olive oil over medium heat. Add the onion and garlic, cooking for 3-4 minutes until softened.
2. Add curry powder, diced tomatoes, coconut milk, lentils, carrots, cauliflower, and 2 cups of water. Bring to a boil.
3. Reduce heat to low, cover, and simmer for 30 minutes, or until lentils are tender.
4. Stir in the spinach and cook for another 5 minutes until wilted.
5. Serve the curry over a bed of cooked brown rice and season with salt and pepper to taste.

NUTRITIONAL BREAKDOWN (PER SERVING):

- Calories: 400
- Carbs: 60g (20% of daily value)
- Protein: 18g (36% of daily value)
- Fiber: 14g (56% of daily value)
- Fats: 12g (18% of daily value)

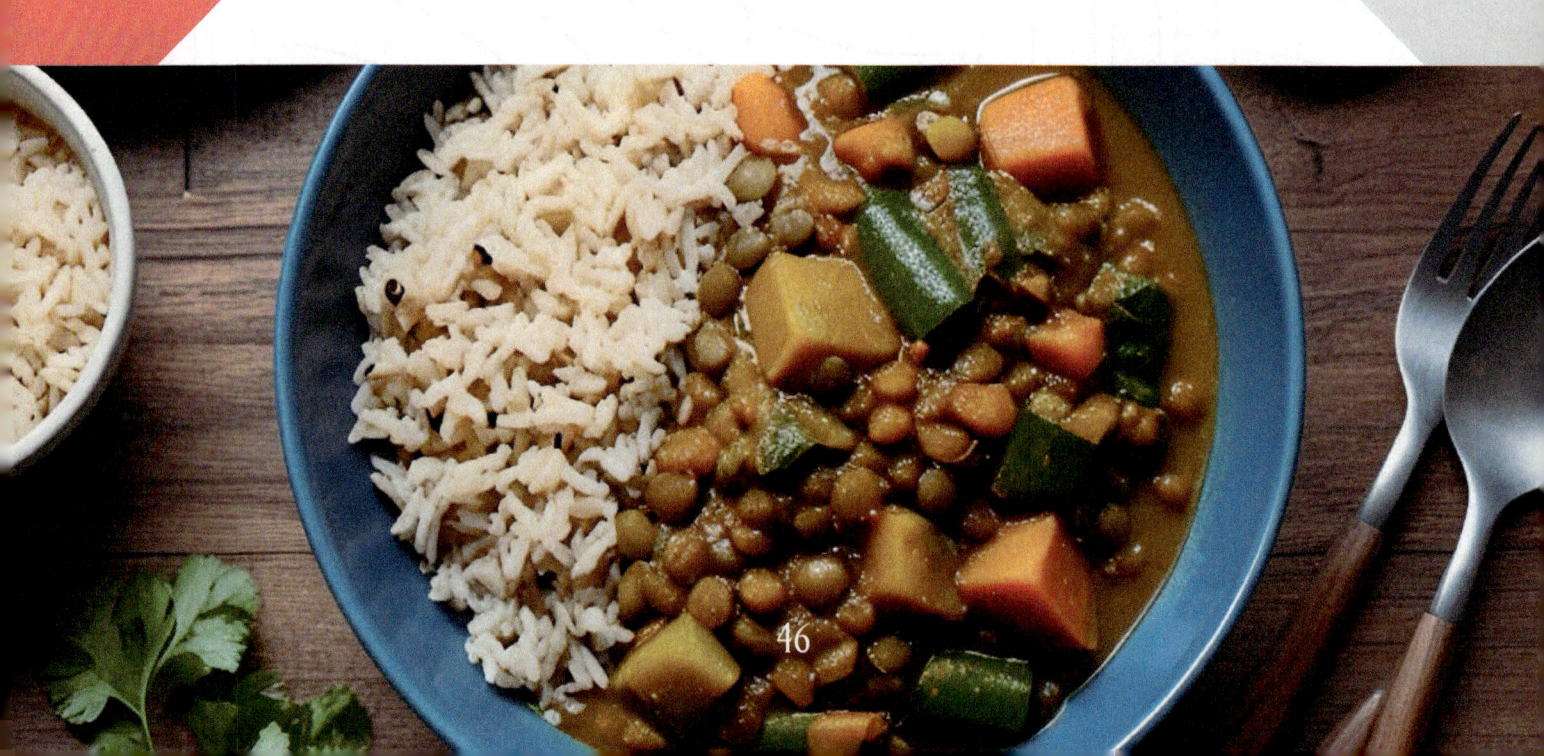

Chapter 6: Appetizers and Salads (Light and Refreshing Bites)

Appetizers and salads often get a bad rap for being boring or too light to satisfy, but that's far from the truth. When prepared with fresh, whole ingredients, these dishes can be bursting with flavor, nutrient-dense, and perfect for managing blood sugar levels. They offer a refreshing break from heavier meals and provide a fun, healthy alternative to store-bought snacks, which are often filled with added sugars and unnecessary preservatives.

Cucumber and Hummus Boats

- Prep Time: 5 minutes
- Cook Time: None
- Total Time: 5 minutes
- Servings: 2

INGREDIENTS :

- 1 large cucumber
- 1/4 cup hummus (store-bought or homemade)
- 1 tbsp fresh parsley, chopped
- 1 tbsp olive oil (optional)
- Salt and pepper, to taste
- 1/2 tsp paprika (optional, for garnish)

NUTRITIONAL BREAKDOWN (PER SERVING):

- Calories: 180
- Carbs: 10g (3% of daily value)
- Protein: 6g (12% of daily value)
- Fiber: 4g (16% of daily value)
- Fats: 14g (22% of daily value)

HOW TO MAKE :

1. Slice the cucumber lengthwise and scoop out the seeds using a spoon to create little "boats."
2. Fill each cucumber boat with a generous amount of hummus.
3. Drizzle with olive oil (if desired) and season with salt and pepper.
4. Garnish with fresh parsley and paprika for an extra pop of flavor.
5. Serve immediately for a fresh, crisp snack or appetizer.

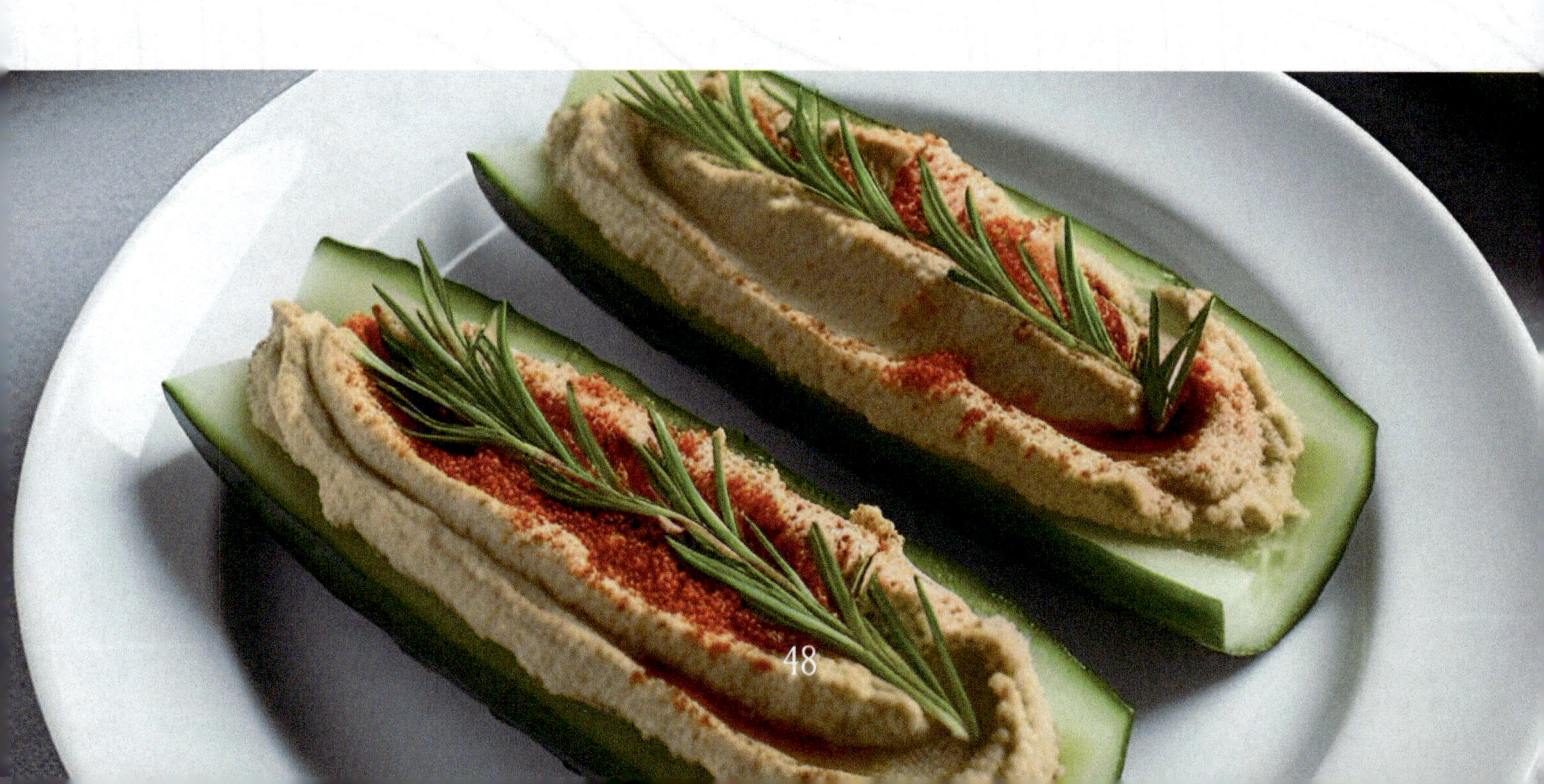

Roasted Red Pepper and Feta Stuffed Mushrooms

- Prep Time: 10 minutes
- Cook Time: 20 minutes
- Total Time: 30 minutes
- Servings: 4

INGREDIENTS :

- 12 large button mushrooms, stems removed
- 1/4 cup roasted red peppers, chopped
- 1/4 cup crumbled feta cheese
- 1 tbsp olive oil
- 1 clove garlic, minced
- 1 tbsp fresh basil, chopped
- Salt and pepper, to taste

NUTRITIONAL BREAKDOWN (PER SERVING):

- Calories: 180
- Carbs: 10g (3% of daily value)
- Protein: 8g (16% of daily value)
- Fiber: 4g (16% of daily value)
- Fats: 14g (22% of daily value)

HOW TO MAKE :

1. Preheat the oven to 375°F (190°C). Place the mushroom caps on a baking sheet lined with parchment paper.
2. In a small bowl, mix the chopped roasted red peppers, feta, garlic, basil, olive oil, salt, and pepper.
3. Spoon the mixture into each mushroom cap, pressing lightly to pack it in.
4. Roast the stuffed mushrooms in the oven for 15-20 minutes, or until the mushrooms are tender and the filling is golden.
5. Serve warm as a savory, bite-sized treat.

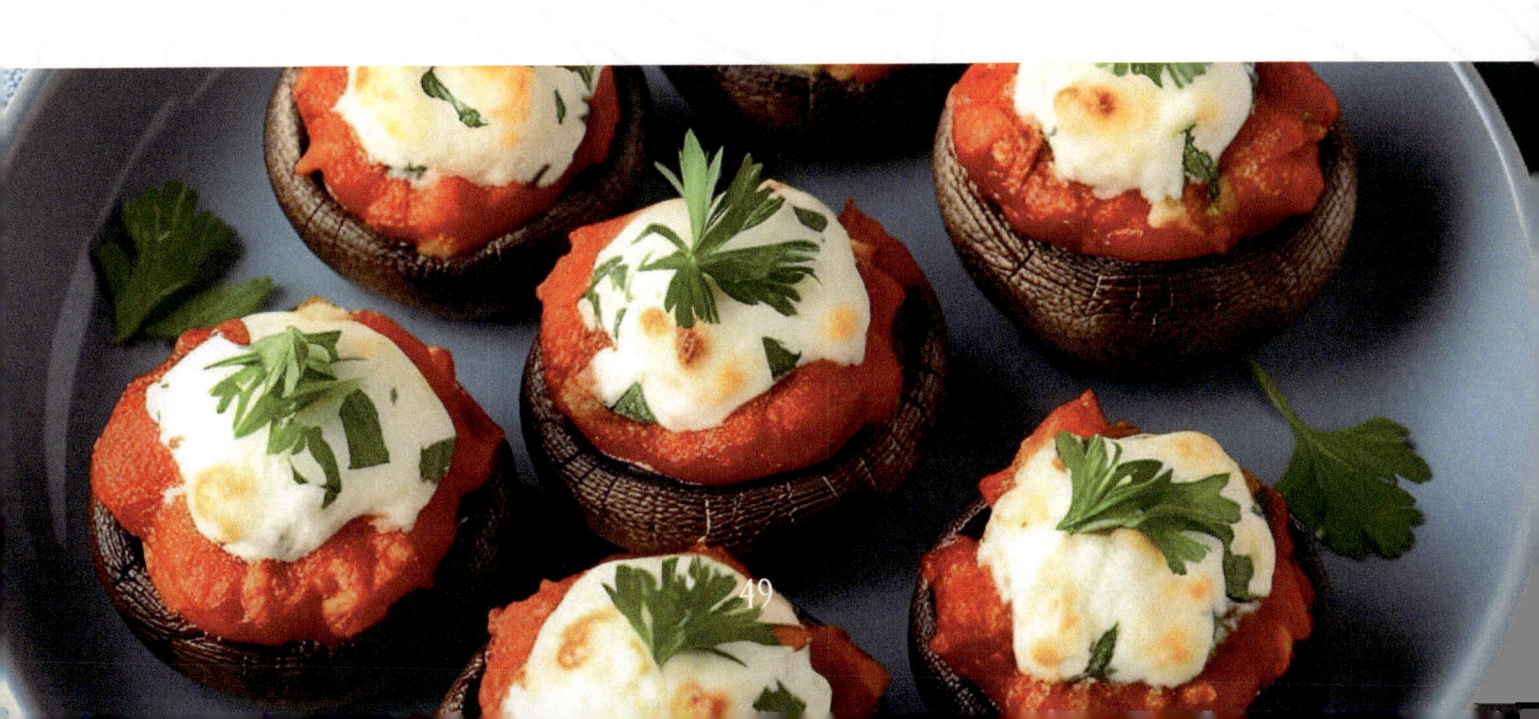

Quinoa Salad with Cucumber, Tomato, and Mint

- Prep Time: 10 minutes
- Cook Time: 15 minutes
- Total Time: 25 minutes
- Servings: 2

INGREDIENTS :

- 1/2 cup quinoa (uncooked)
- 1 cucumber, diced
- 1 cup cherry tomatoes, halved
- 1/4 cup fresh mint, chopped
- 1 tbsp olive oil
- 1 tbsp lemon juice
- Salt and pepper, to taste

NUTRITIONAL BREAKDOWN (PER SERVING):

- Calories: 250
- Carbs: 38g (13% of daily value)
- Protein: 8g (16% of daily value)
- Fiber: 6g (24% of daily value)
- Fats: 10g (15% of daily value)

HOW TO MAKE :

1. Rinse the quinoa thoroughly, then cook it according to package instructions (usually 10-15 minutes).
2. Once the quinoa is cooked and cooled, transfer it to a large bowl.
3. Add the diced cucumber, cherry tomatoes, and chopped mint to the quinoa. Toss to combine.
4. Drizzle with olive oil and lemon juice, then season with salt and pepper to taste.
5. Serve chilled or at room temperature for a refreshing, light salad.

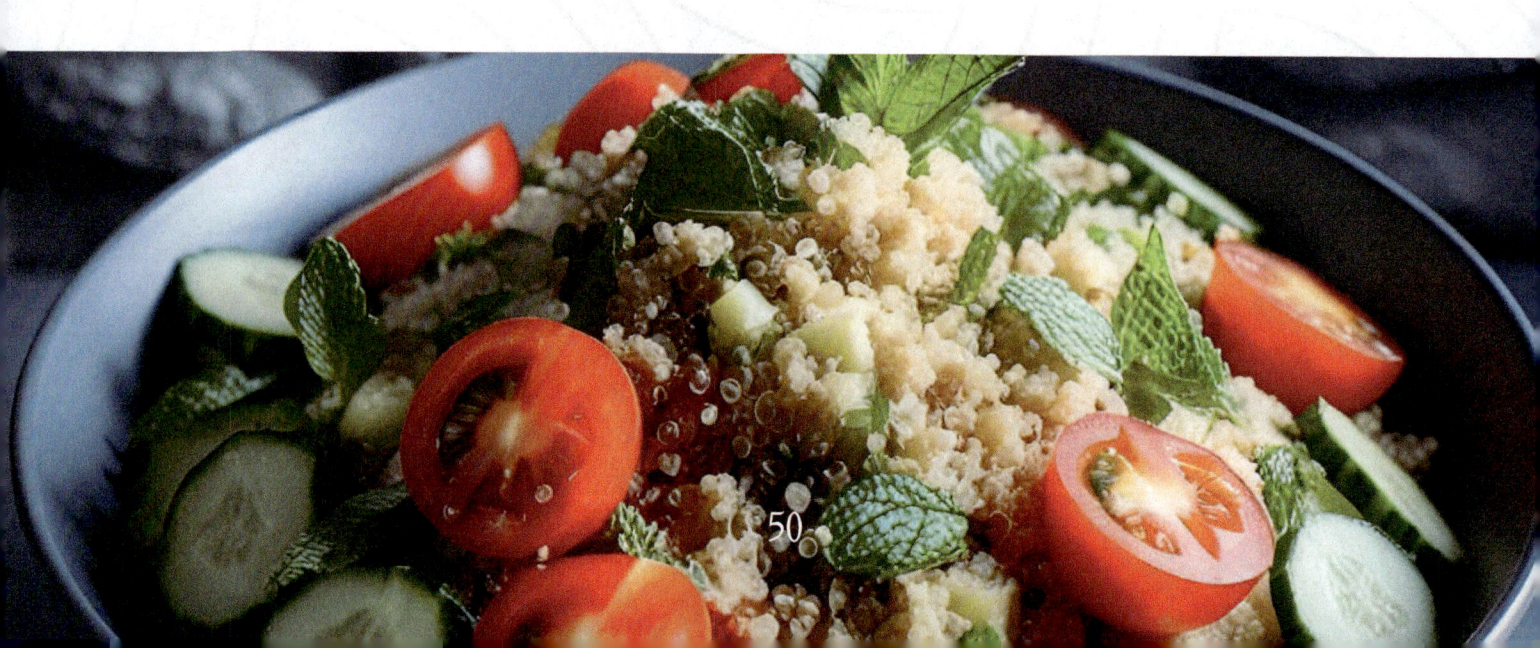

Grilled Veggie Skewers with Lemon-Tahini Dressing

- Prep Time: 15 minutes
- Cook Time: 10 minutes
- Total Time: 25 minutes
- Servings: 2

INGREDIENTS :

- 1 zucchini, sliced into rounds
- 1 red bell pepper, cut into chunks
- 1/2 red onion, cut into chunks
- 1 tbsp olive oil
- Salt and pepper, to taste

FOR THE LEMON-TAHINI DRESSING

- 2 tbsp tahini
- 1 tbsp lemon juice
- 1 tsp olive oil
- 1/2 tsp garlic powder
- Salt and pepper, to taste

HOW TO MAKE :

1. Preheat the grill or grill pan over medium heat.
2. Thread the zucchini, bell pepper, and red onion onto skewers. Drizzle with olive oil and season with salt and pepper.
3. Grill the veggie skewers for 5-7 minutes on each side, or until the vegetables are tender and slightly charred.
4. While the vegetables are grilling, whisk together tahini, lemon juice, olive oil, garlic powder, salt, and pepper in a small bowl to create the dressing.
5. Drizzle the lemon-tahini dressing over the grilled vegetables and serve immediately.

NUTRITIONAL BREAKDOWN (PER SERVING):

- Calories: 250
- Carbs: 20g (7% of daily value)
- Protein: 6g (12% of daily value)
- Fiber: 6g (24% of daily value)
- Fats: 18g (28% of daily value)

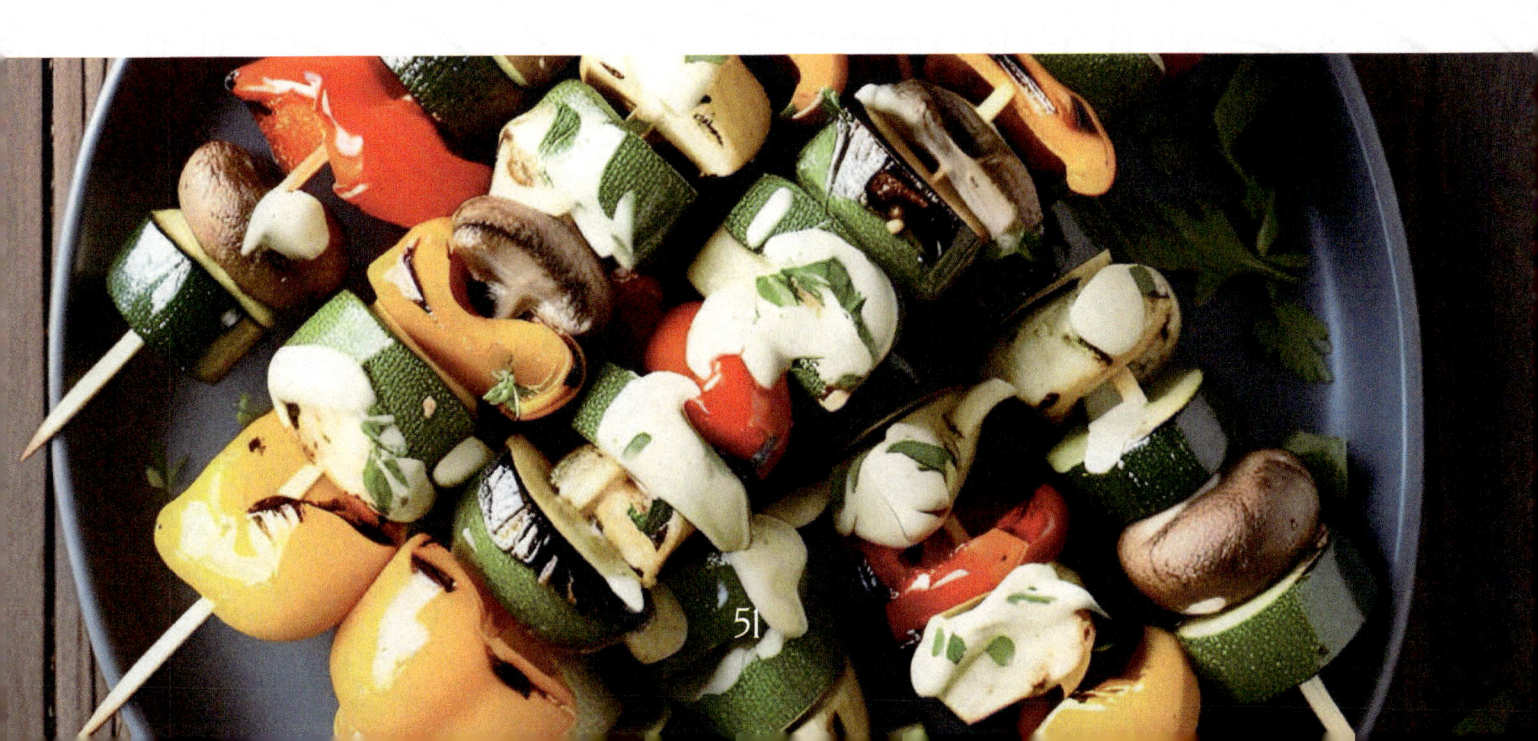

Sweet Potato and Kale Salad with Balsamic Dressing

- Prep Time: 10 minutes
- Cook Time: 20 minutes
- Total Time: 30 minutes
- Servings: 2

INGREDIENTS :

- 1 medium sweet potato, cubed
- 1 tbsp olive oil
- 2 cups kale, chopped
- 1/4 cup dried cranberries (unsweetened)
- 1/4 cup walnuts, chopped

FOR THE LEMON-TAHINI DRESSING

- 2 tbsp balsamic vinegar
- 1 tbsp olive oil
- 1 tsp Dijon mustard
- Salt and pepper, to taste

NUTRITIONAL BREAKDOWN (PER SERVING):

- Calories: 350
- Carbs: 45g (15% of daily value)
- Protein: 8g (16% of daily value)
- Fiber: 10g (40% of daily value)
- Fats: 18g (28% of daily value)

HOW TO MAKE :

1. Preheat the oven to 400°F (200°C). Toss the sweet potato cubes with olive oil and season with salt and pepper. Roast for 20 minutes, or until tender.
2. While the sweet potatoes are roasting, massage the kale with a bit of olive oil and salt to soften it.
3. Once the sweet potatoes are done, allow them to cool slightly before combining them with the kale, dried cranberries, and walnuts in a large bowl.
4. Whisk together balsamic vinegar, olive oil, Dijon mustard, salt, and pepper for the dressing.
5. Drizzle the dressing over the salad, toss to combine, and serve immediately.

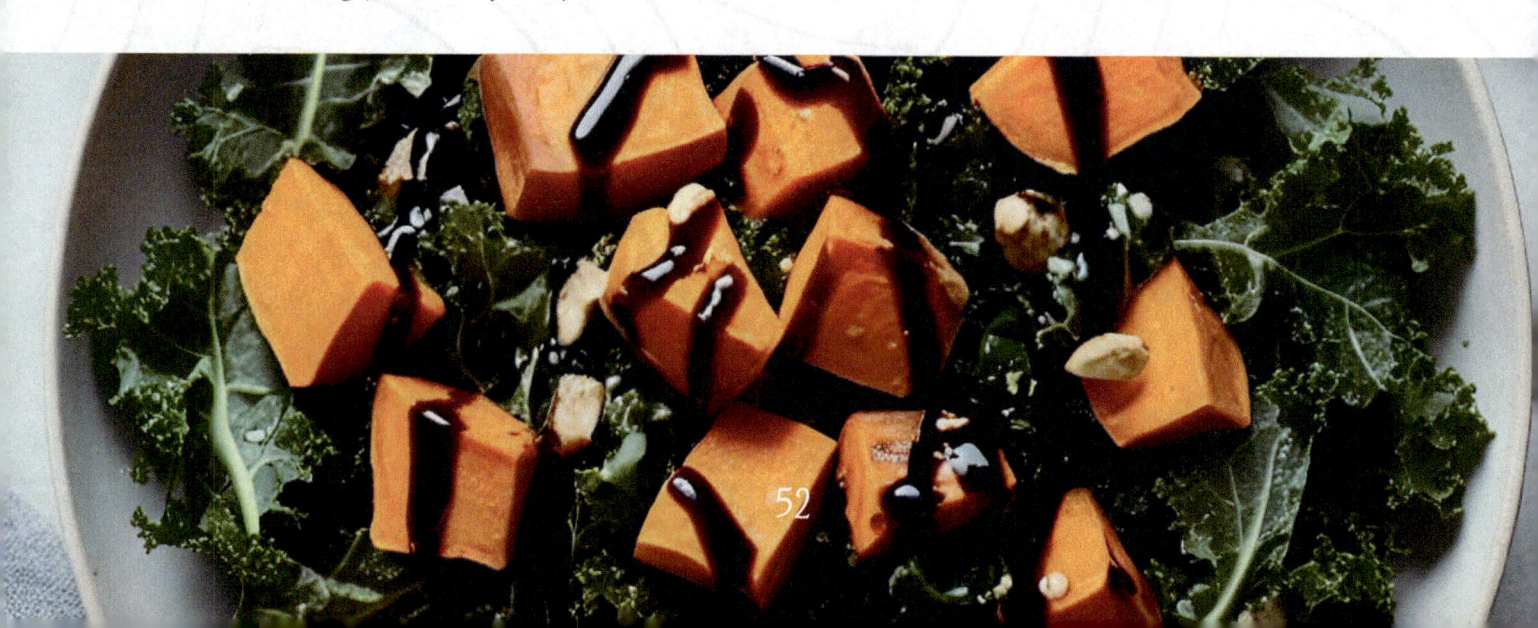

Mediterranean Chickpea Salad with Olives and Feta

- Prep Time: 10 minutes
- Cook Time: None
- Total Time: 10 minutes
- Servings: 2

INGREDIENTS :

- 1 can (15 oz) chickpeas, drained and rinsed
- 1/4 cup Kalamata olives, pitted and chopped
- 1/4 cup feta cheese, crumbled
- 1/2 cucumber, diced
- 1/2 red onion, finely chopped
- 1/2 cup cherry tomatoes, halved
- 1 tbsp olive oil
- 1 tbsp red wine vinegar
- 1 tsp dried oregano
- Salt and pepper, to taste

HOW TO MAKE :

1. In a large bowl, combine the chickpeas, olives, feta, cucumber, red onion, and cherry tomatoes.
2. In a small bowl, whisk together the olive oil, red wine vinegar, oregano, salt, and pepper
3. Pour the dressing over the salad and toss to combine.
4. Serve immediately or refrigerate for a few hours for the flavors to meld.

NUTRITIONAL BREAKDOWN (PER SERVING):

- Calories: 300
- Carbs: 30g (10% of daily value)
- Protein: 10g (20% of daily value)
- Fiber: 8g (32% of daily value)
- Fats: 18g (28% of daily value)

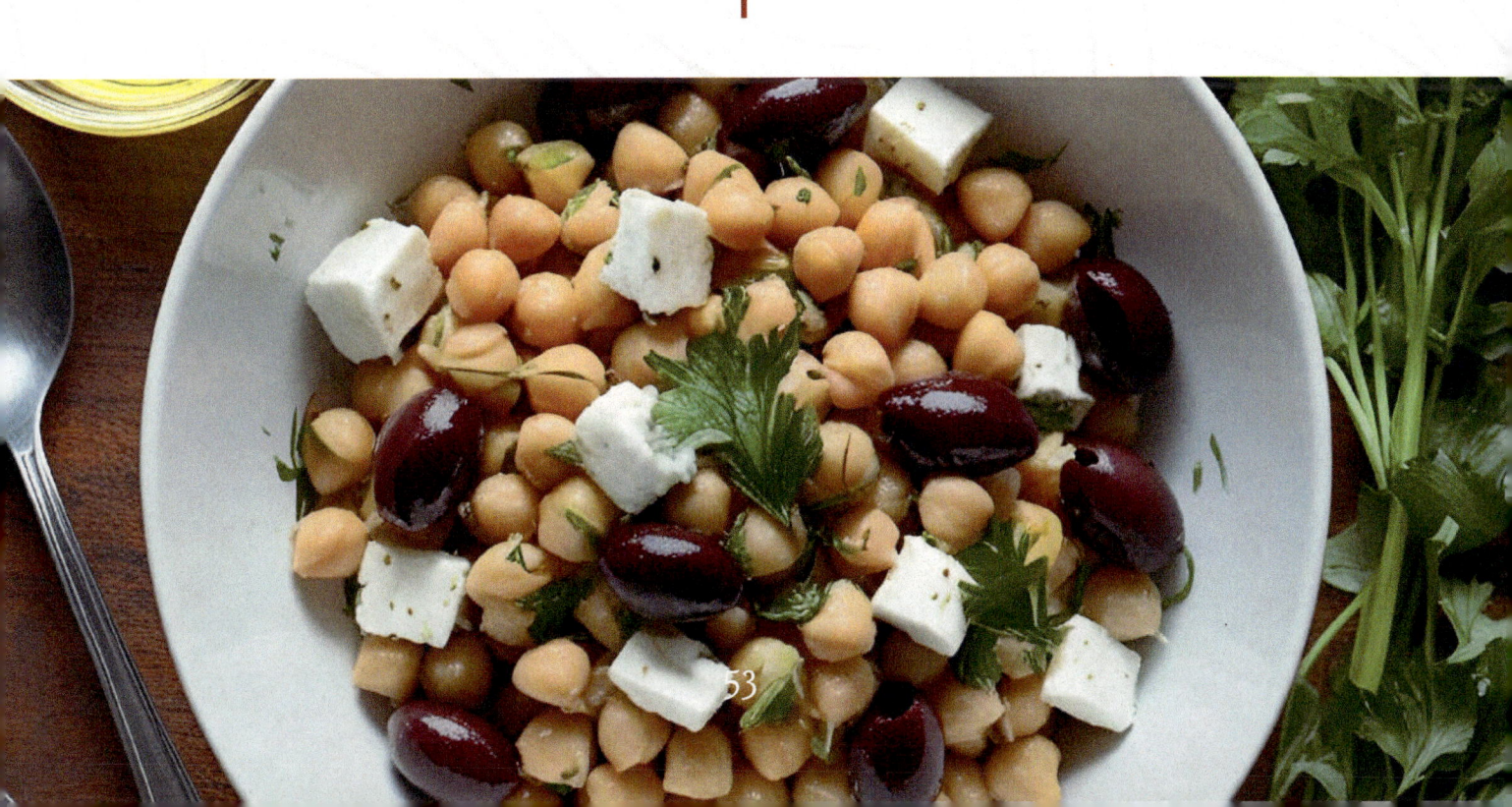

Spinach and Strawberry Salad with Walnuts

- Prep Time: 5 minutes
- Cook Time: None
- Total Time: 5 minutes
- Servings: 2

INGREDIENTS :

- 3 cups fresh spinach
- 1/2 cup fresh strawberries, sliced
- 1/4 cup walnuts, chopped
- 1/4 cup goat cheese (optional)

FOR THE DRESSING:

- 1 tbsp balsamic vinegar
- 1 tsp honey or stevia
- 1 tbsp olive oil
- Salt and pepper, to taste

HOW TO MAKE :

1. In a large bowl, combine the spinach, strawberries, and walnuts.
2. For the dressing, whisk together the balsamic vinegar, honey (or stevia), olive oil, salt, and pepper.
3. Drizzle the dressing over the salad and toss gently to coat.
4. Top with goat cheese, if desired, and serve immediately.

NUTRITIONAL BREAKDOWN (PER SERVING):

- Calories: 220
- Protein: 6g (12% of daily intake)
- Fat: 14g (21% of daily intake)
- Carbs: 18g (6% of daily intake)
- Fiber: 3g (12% of daily intake)
- Vitamin E: 10% of daily intake (from almond butter)

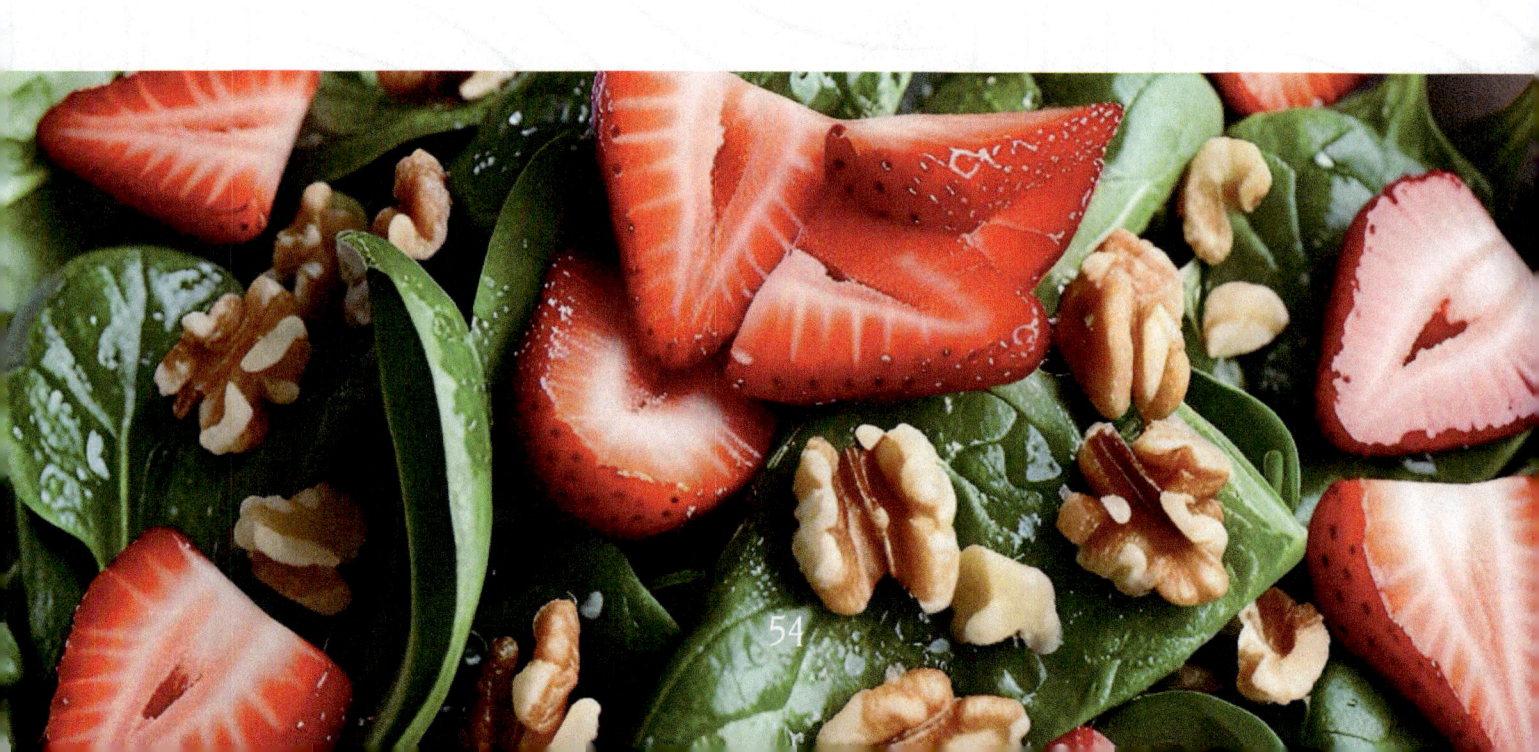

Avocado, Tomato, and Cucumber Salad with Lime Dressing

- Prep Time: 5 minutes
- Cook Time: None
- Total Time: 5 minutes
- Servings: 2

INGREDIENTS :

- 1 avocado, diced
- 1/2 cucumber, sliced
- 1/2 cup cherry tomatoes, halved
- 1 tbsp fresh cilantro, chopped

FOR THE DRESSING:

- 1 tbsp lime juice
- 1 tbsp olive oil
- 1/2 tsp cumin
- Salt and pepper, to taste

HOW TO MAKE :

1. In a bowl, combine the avocado, cucumber, cherry tomatoes, and cilantro.
2. In a small bowl, whisk together the lime juice, olive oil, cumin, salt, and pepper.
3. Drizzle the dressing over the salad and toss gently to combine.
4. Serve immediately for a refreshing, light snack or side dish.

NUTRITIONAL BREAKDOWN (PER SERVING):

- Calories: 200
- Carbs: 12g (4% of daily value)
- Protein: 3g (6% of daily value)
- Fiber: 8g (32% of daily value)
- Fats: 18g (28% of daily value)

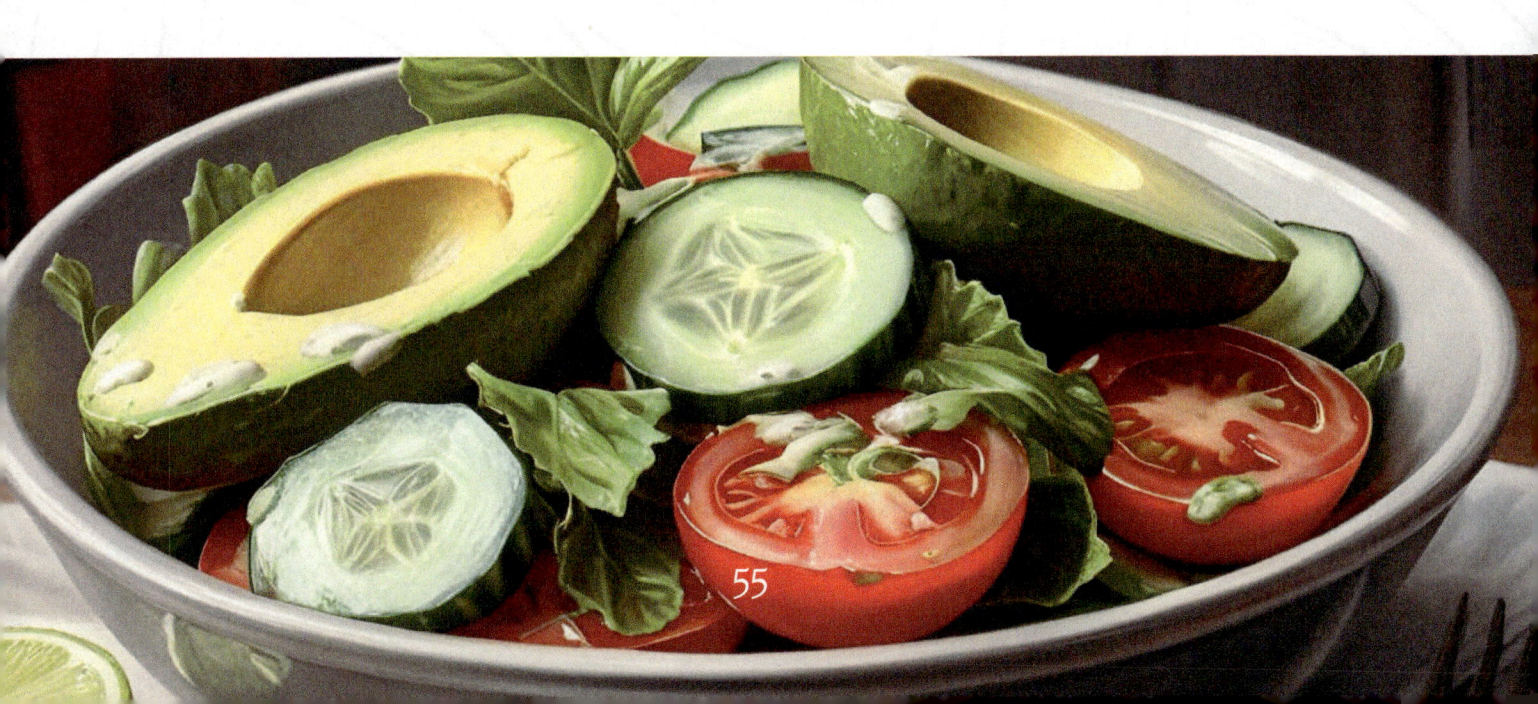

Chapter 7: Soups and Stews (Hearty and Nutritious)

When it comes to comfort food that nourishes the body while stabilizing blood sugar, few meals can compare to a warm bowl of soup or stew. These dishes are not only satisfying but also packed with nutrients that support digestion, energy levels, and overall well-being. Soups and stews are an excellent way to incorporate a variety of vegetables, legumes, and whole grains, which are key to managing blood sugar effectively.

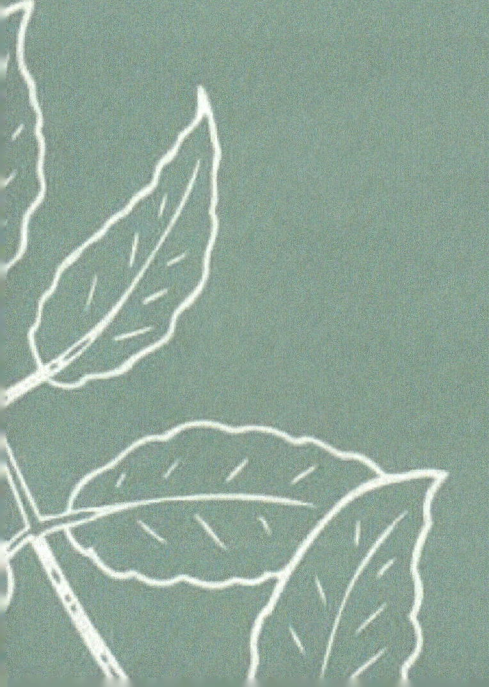

Lentil Soup with Spinach and Carrots

- Prep Time: 10 minutes
- Cook Time: 30 minutes
- Total Time: 40 minutes
- Servings: 4

INGREDIENTS :

- 1 cup dried lentils, rinsed
- 1 tbsp olive oil
- 1 small onion, chopped
- 2 carrots, peeled and diced
- 2 cloves garlic, minced
- 4 cups vegetable broth (low-sodium)
- 2 cups fresh spinach (or frozen)
- 1 tsp cumin
- 1/2 tsp turmeric
- Salt and pepper, to taste
- 1 tbsp lemon juice (optional)

NUTRITIONAL BREAKDOWN (PER SERVING):

- Calories: 280
- Carbs: 45g (15% of daily value)
- Protein: 18g (36% of daily value)
- Fiber: 15g (60% of daily value)
- Fats: 7g (11% of daily value)

HOW TO MAKE :

1. Heat olive oil in a large pot over medium heat. Add the onion and carrots and cook for 5-7 minutes until softened.
2. Add garlic, cumin, and turmeric, and cook for another minute until fragrant.
3. Stir in the lentils and vegetable broth. Bring to a boil, then reduce heat to low and simmer, covered, for 25-30 minutes, or until the lentils are tender.
4. Add the spinach and cook for another 3-5 minutes until wilted.
5. Stir in lemon juice, if desired, and season with salt and pepper. Serve warm.

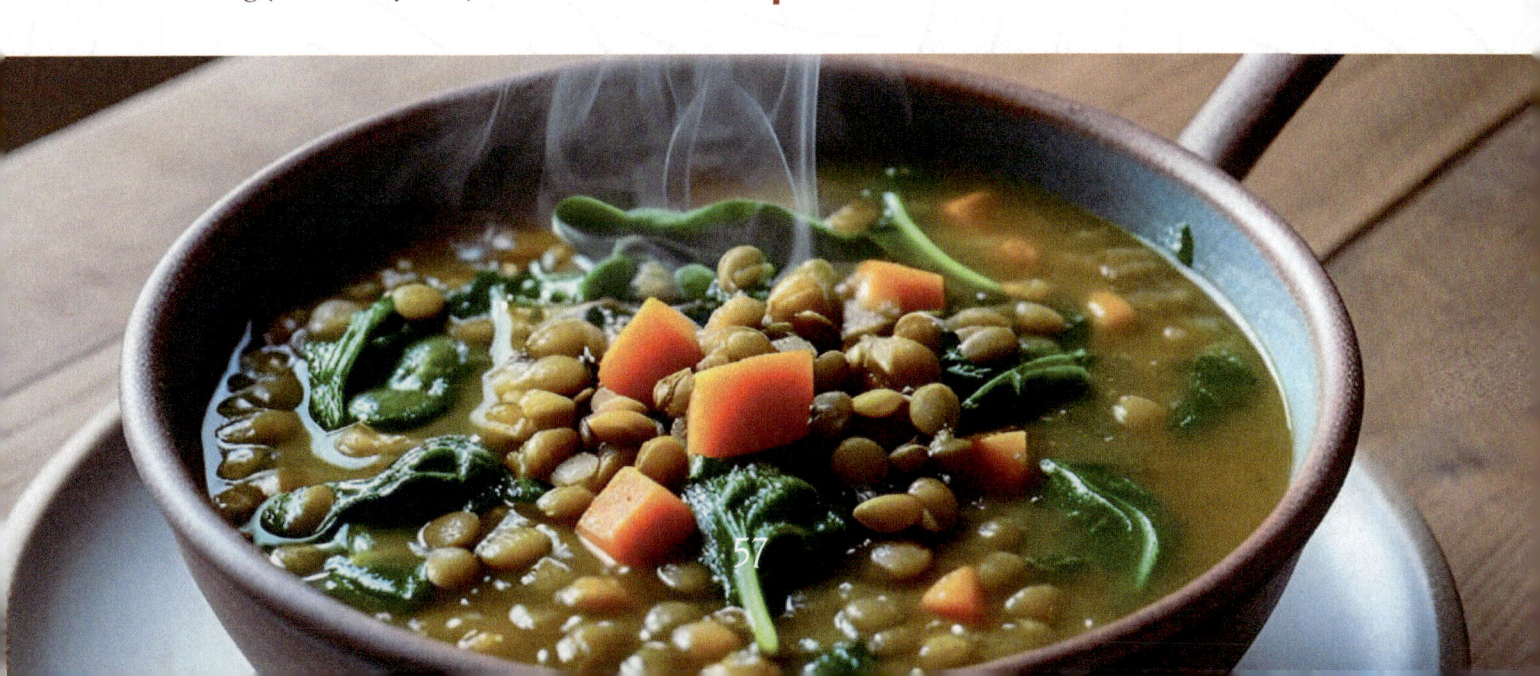

Tomato Basil Soup with a Touch of Coconut Milk

- Prep Time: 5 minutes
- Cook Time: 25 minutes
- Total Time: 30 minutes
- Servings: 4

INGREDIENTS :

- 2 cups canned diced tomatoes (no added sugar)
- 1 tbsp olive oil
- 1 small onion, chopped
- 2 cloves garlic, minced
- 1 cup unsweetened coconut milk
- 2 cups vegetable broth (low-sodium)
- 1/4 cup fresh basil, chopped
- Salt and pepper, to taste
- 1/2 tsp red pepper flakes (optional)

NUTRITIONAL BREAKDOWN (PER SERVING):

- Calories: 220
- Carbs: 18g (6% of daily value)
- Protein: 3g (6% of daily value)
- Fiber: 6g (24% of daily value)
- Fats: 15g (23% of daily value)

HOW TO MAKE :

1. Heat olive oil in a large pot over medium heat. Add the onion and cook for 5-7 minutes, until softened.
2. Add garlic and cook for another minute until fragrant.
3. Stir in the diced tomatoes, coconut milk, vegetable broth, and red pepper flakes (if using). Bring to a simmer and cook for 20 minutes, stirring occasionally.
4. Once the soup has thickened slightly, use an immersion blender to puree the soup to your desired consistency (or transfer to a blender).
5. Stir in fresh basil and season with salt and pepper. Serve warm.

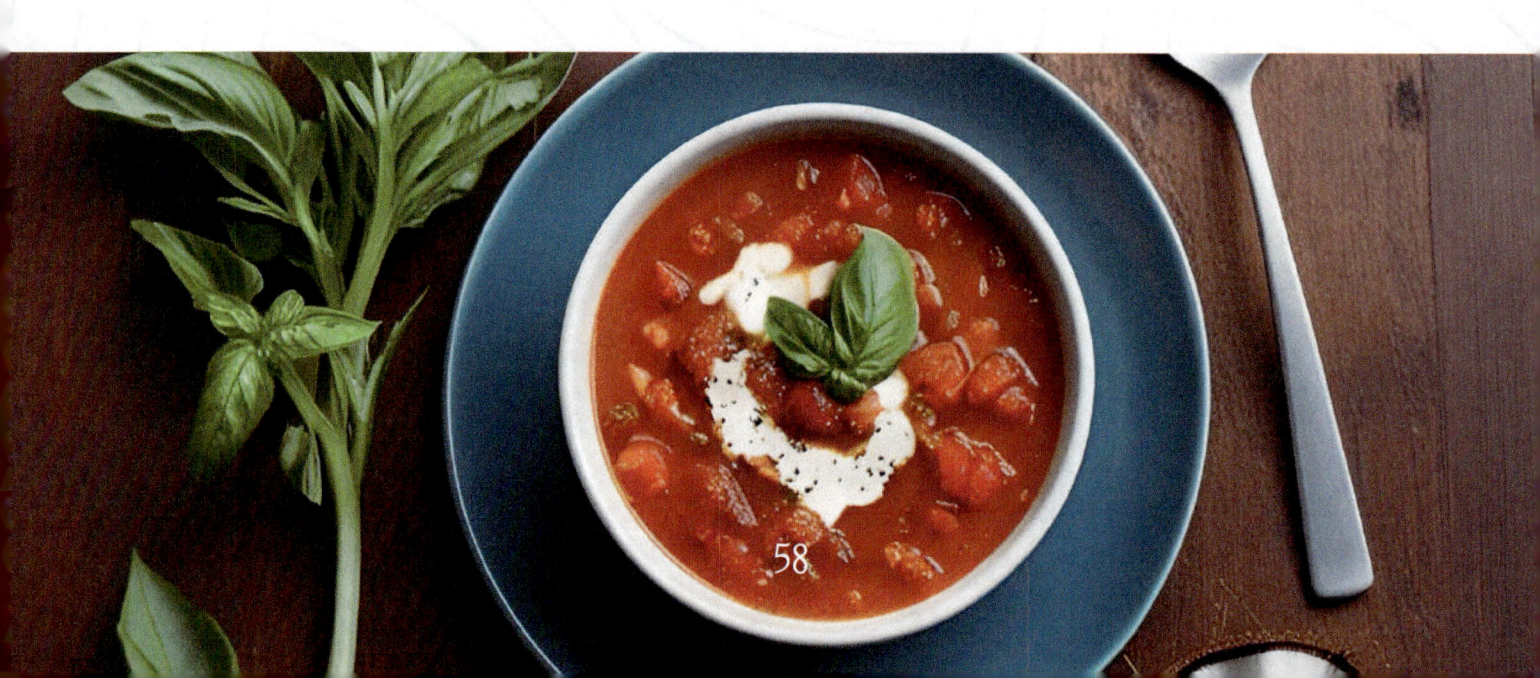

Butternut Squash and Kale Soup

- Prep Time: 10 minutes
- Cook Time: 30 minutes
- Total Time: 40 minutes
- Servings: 4

INGREDIENTS :

- 1 small butternut squash, peeled, seeded, and cubed
- 1 tbsp olive oil
- 1 small onion, chopped
- 2 cloves garlic, minced
- 4 cups vegetable broth (low-sodium)
- 2 cups kale, chopped
- 1/2 tsp cinnamon
- 1/4 tsp nutmeg
- Salt and pepper, to taste
- 1 tbsp apple cider vinegar (optional)

NUTRITIONAL BREAKDOWN (PER SERVING):

- Calories: 250
- Carbs: 45g (15% of daily value)
- Protein: 5g (10% of daily value)
- Fiber: 10g (40% of daily value)
- Fats: 8g (12% of daily value)

HOW TO MAKE :

1. Heat olive oil in a large pot over medium heat. Add the onion and garlic and cook for 5 minutes, until softened.
2. Stir in the butternut squash, cinnamon, and nutmeg, and cook for 3-4 minutes.
3. Add vegetable broth and bring to a simmer. Cook for 20-25 minutes, until the squash is tender.
4. Use an immersion blender to puree the soup, or transfer to a blender in batches. Return the soup to the pot.
5. Stir in the kale and cook for another 5-7 minutes, until wilted.
6. Add apple cider vinegar, if desired, and season with salt and pepper to taste. Serve warm.

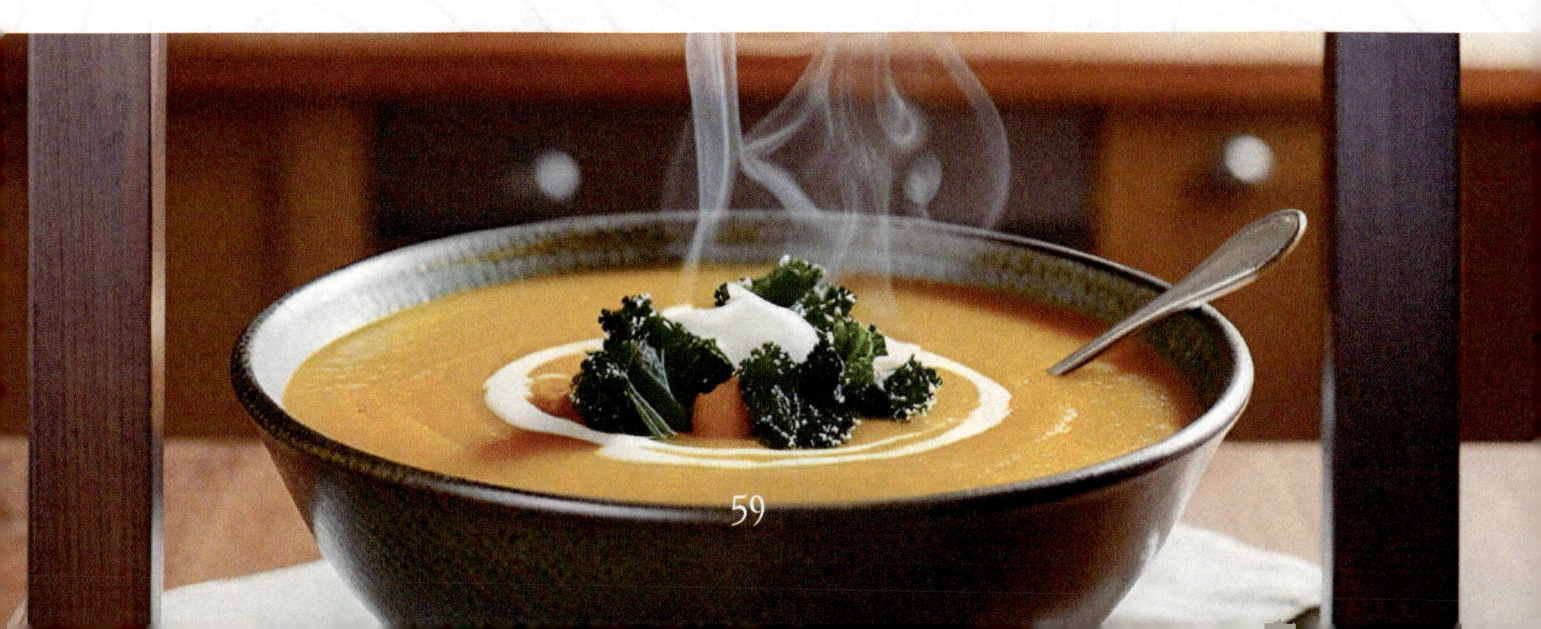

Chickpea and Vegetable Stew

- Prep Time: 10 minutes
- Cook Time: 30 minutes
- Total Time: 40 minutes
- Servings: 4

INGREDIENTS :

- 1 can (15 oz) chickpeas, drained and rinsed
- 1 tbsp olive oil
- 1 small onion, chopped
- 2 carrots, peeled and diced
- 1 zucchini, diced
- 1/2 cup diced tomatoes (canned or fresh)
- 4 cups vegetable broth (low-sodium)
- 1 tsp cumin
- 1/2 tsp coriander
- 1/4 tsp turmeric
- Salt and pepper, to taste
- 1 tbsp fresh parsley, chopped (optional)

HOW TO MAKE :

1. Heat olive oil in a large pot over medium heat. Add the onion and cook for 5 minutes, until softened.
2. Add the carrots and zucchini, and cook for 5 more minutes, stirring occasionally.
3. Stir in the chickpeas, diced tomatoes, vegetable broth, cumin, coriander, and turmeric. Bring to a boil, then reduce heat and simmer for 20 minutes.
4. Season with salt and pepper, and stir in fresh parsley before serving.

NUTRITIONAL BREAKDOWN (PER SERVING):

- Calories: 290
- Carbs: 45g (15% of daily value)
- Protein: 12g (24% of daily value)
- Fiber: 12g (48% of daily value)
- Fats: 8g (12% of daily value)

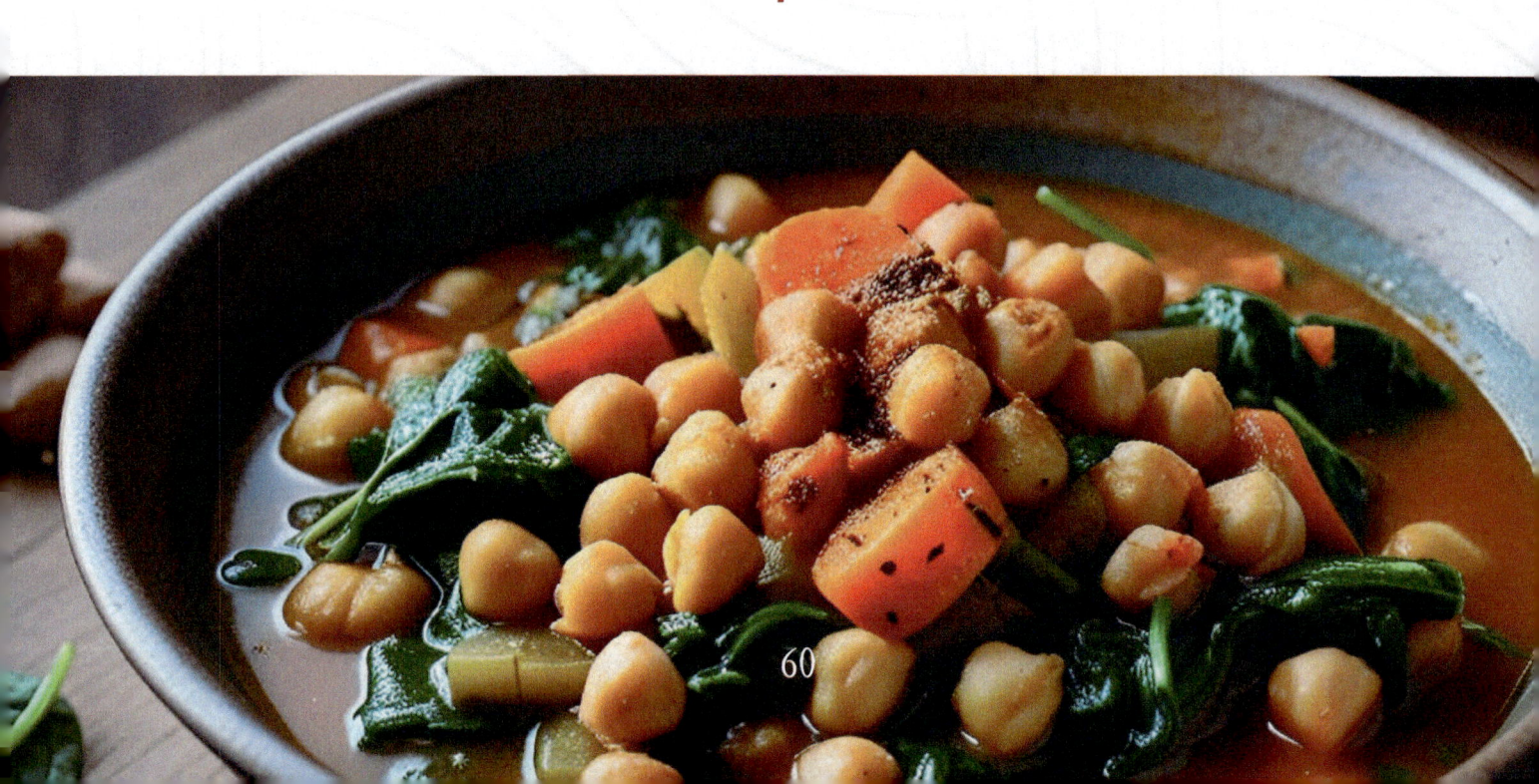

Mushroom Barley Soup

- Prep Time: 10 minutes
- Cook Time: 30 minutes
- Total Time: 40 minutes
- Servings: 4

INGREDIENTS :

- 1 tbsp olive oil
- 1 small onion, chopped
- 2 cloves garlic, minced
- 2 cups mushrooms, sliced
- 1/2 cup pearl barley
- 4 cups vegetable broth (low-sodium)
- 1/2 tsp thyme
- 1/2 tsp rosemary
- Salt and pepper, to taste
- 1 tbsp fresh parsley, chopped (optional)

NUTRITIONAL BREAKDOWN (PER SERVING):

- Calories: 220
- Carbs: 40g (13% of daily value)
- Protein: 8g (16% of daily value)
- Fiber: 8g (32% of daily value)
- Fats: 5g (8% of daily value)

HOW TO MAKE :

1. Heat olive oil in a large pot over medium heat. Add the onion and garlic, and cook for 3-4 minutes until softened.
2. Add the mushrooms and cook for another 5 minutes, until they release their moisture and begin to brown.
3. Stir in the pearl barley, vegetable broth, thyme, rosemary, salt, and pepper. Bring to a boil, then reduce the heat to low and simmer, covered, for 25-30 minutes, or until the barley is tender.
4. Garnish with fresh parsley and serve warm.

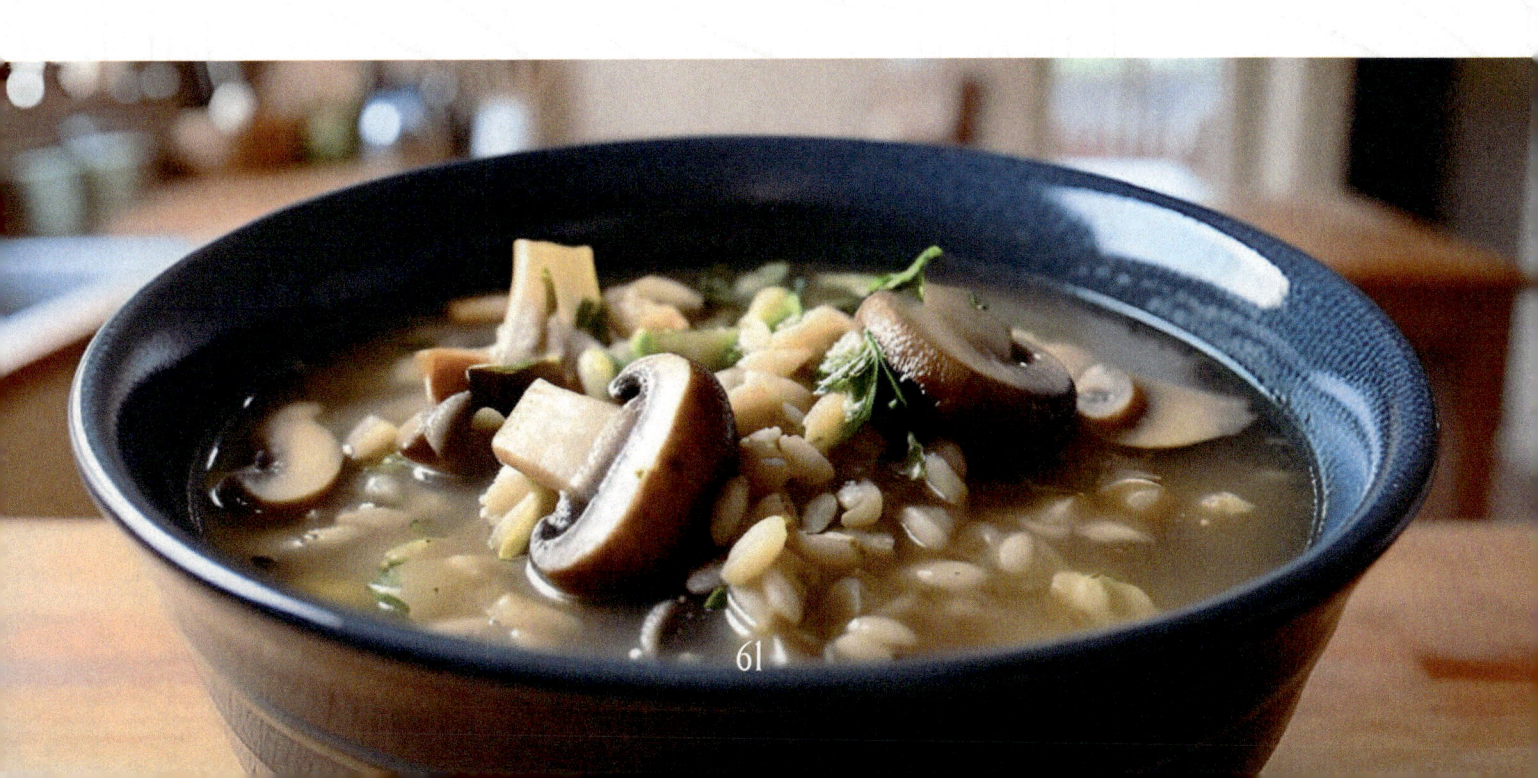

Spicy Black Bean Soup with Lime

- Prep Time: 10 minutes
- Cook Time: 25 minutes
- Total Time: 35 minutes
- Servings: 4

INGREDIENTS :

- 2 cans (15 oz each) black beans, drained and rinsed
- 1 tbsp olive oil
- 1 small onion, chopped
- 2 cloves garlic, minced
- 1 red bell pepper, chopped
- 1 tsp cumin
- 1/2 tsp chili powder
- 1/4 tsp cayenne pepper (adjust to spice preference)
- 4 cups vegetable broth (low-sodium)
- 1 tbsp lime juice
- Salt and pepper, to taste
- Fresh cilantro, for garnish

NUTRITIONAL BREAKDOWN (PER SERVING):

- Calories: 250
- Carbs: 40g (13% of daily value)
- Protein: 15g (30% of daily value)
- Fiber: 12g (48% of daily value)
- Fats: 6g (9% of daily value)

HOW TO MAKE :

1. Heat olive oil in a large pot over medium heat. Add the onion, garlic, and bell pepper, and cook for 5 minutes, until softened.
2. Stir in the cumin, chili powder, cayenne pepper, and cook for another minute until fragrant.
3. Add the black beans and vegetable broth, and bring to a simmer. Cook for 15-20 minutes, allowing the flavors to meld together.
4. Use an immersion blender to puree part of the soup for a creamier texture (or transfer to a blender in batches). Leave some beans whole for texture.
5. Stir in the lime juice and season with salt and pepper.
6. Serve with a garnish of fresh cilantro and a squeeze of extra lime juice, if desired.

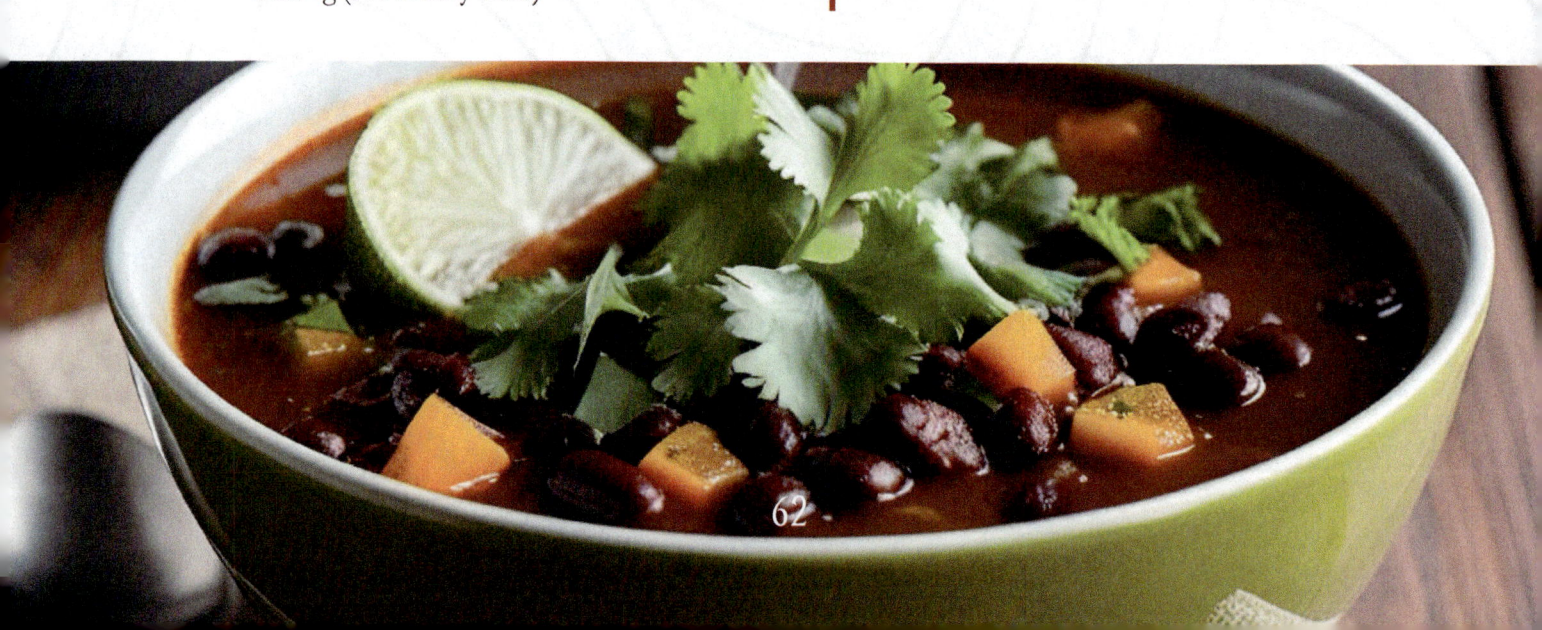

Cauliflower and Leek Soup

- Prep Time: 10 minutes
- Cook Time: 30 minutes
- Total Time: 40 minutes
- Servings: 4

INGREDIENTS :

- 1 tbsp olive oil
- 1 leek, cleaned and chopped
- 1 small onion, chopped
- 2 cloves garlic, minced
- 1 head cauliflower, chopped into florets
- 4 cups vegetable broth (low-sodium)
- 1/2 tsp turmeric
- Salt and pepper, to taste
- 1/2 cup unsweetened coconut milk (optional, for creaminess)

NUTRITIONAL BREAKDOWN (PER SERVING):

- Calories: 200
- Carbs: 25g (8% of daily value)
- Protein: 6g (12% of daily value)
- Fiber: 8g (32% of daily value)
- Fats: 8g (12% of daily value)

HOW TO MAKE :

1. Heat olive oil in a large pot over medium heat. Add the leek, onion, and garlic, and cook for 5-7 minutes until softened.
2. Add the cauliflower florets and cook for another 5 minutes.
3. Pour in the vegetable broth and turmeric. Bring to a boil, then reduce the heat and simmer for 20 minutes, or until the cauliflower is tender.
4. Use an immersion blender to puree the soup to your desired texture (smooth or chunky).
5. Stir in coconut milk, if using, and season with salt and pepper.
6. Serve warm, garnished with fresh herbs or a sprinkle of extra turmeric for a vibrant touch.

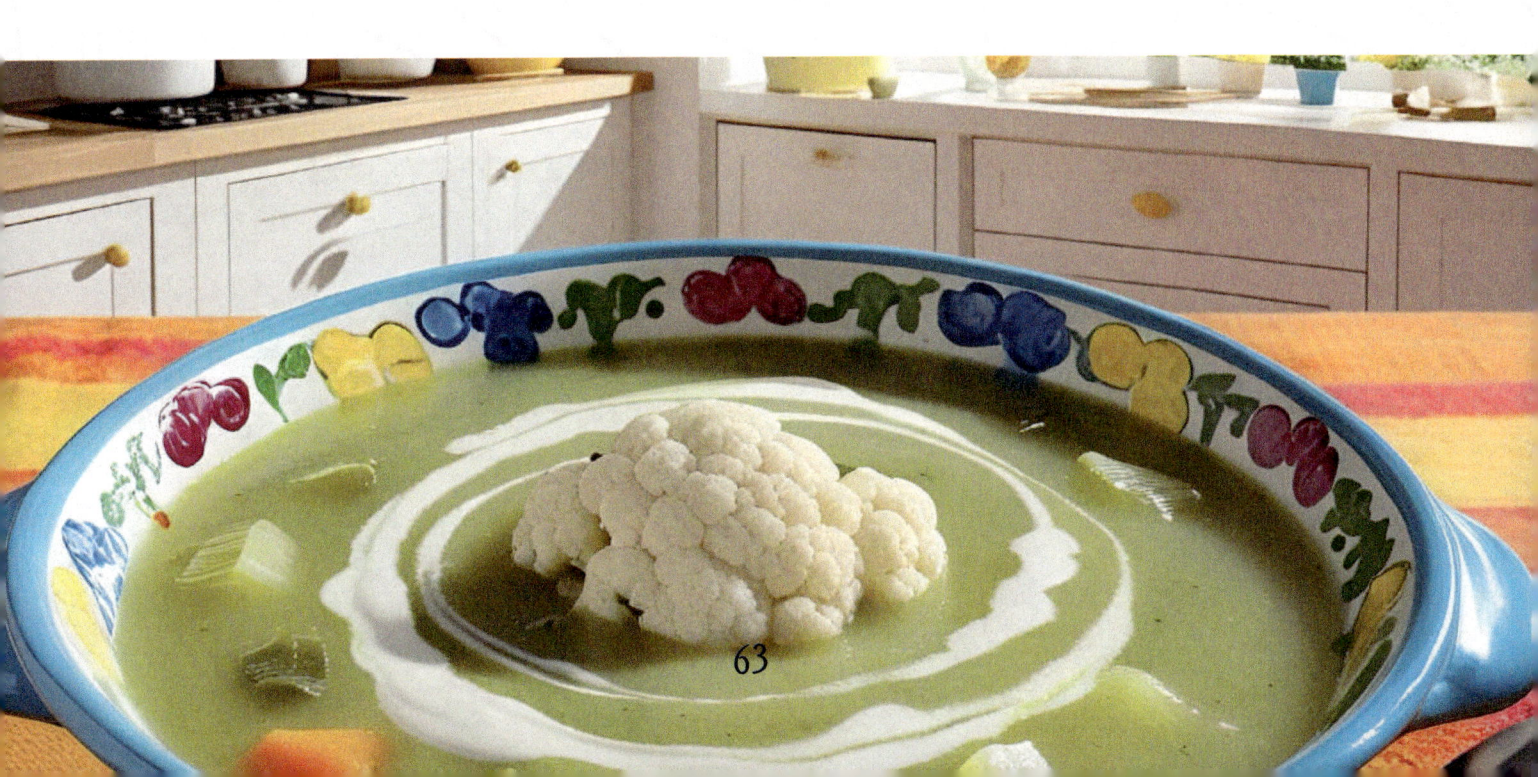

Carrot and Ginger Soup

- Prep Time: 10 minutes
- Cook Time: 30 minutes
- Total Time: 40 minutes
- Servings: 4

INGREDIENTS :

- 1 tbsp olive oil
- 1 small onion, chopped
- 4 large carrots, peeled and chopped
- 2 cloves garlic, minced
- 1-inch piece fresh ginger, peeled and grated
- 4 cups vegetable broth (low-sodium)
- 1/2 tsp cumin
- Salt and pepper, to taste
- 1/4 cup coconut milk (optional, for creaminess)

HOW TO MAKE :

1. Heat olive oil in a large pot over medium heat. Add the onion and garlic, cooking for 5 minutes until softened.
2. Stir in the grated ginger, cumin, and carrots. Cook for an additional 3-4 minutes.
3. Pour in the vegetable broth and bring to a boil. Reduce heat and simmer for 20-25 minutes, until the carrots are tender.
4. Use an immersion blender to puree the soup to your desired consistency.
5. Stir in coconut milk (if desired), season with salt and pepper, and serve warm.

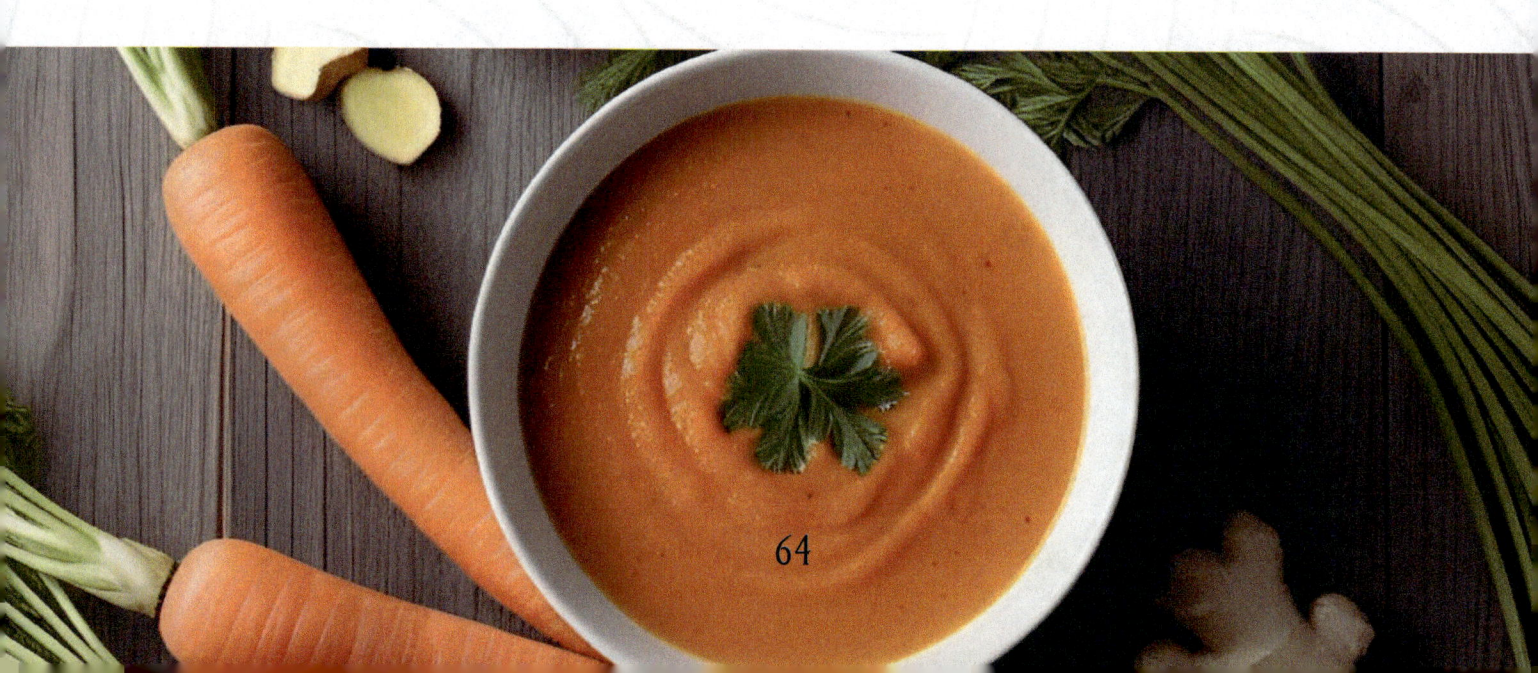

NUTRITIONAL BREAKDOWN (PER SERVING):

- Calories: 180
- Carbs: 30g (10% of daily value)
- Protein: 4g (8% of daily value)
- Fiber: 9g (36% of daily value)
- Fats: 7g (10% of daily value)

Chapter 8: Fish and Seafood (Lean Proteins with Omega-3 Power)

Fish and seafood are among the best sources of lean protein that help maintain stable blood sugar levels while providing essential nutrients like omega-3 fatty acids, which support heart health and reduce inflammation. For anyone managing prediabetes, including fatty fish like salmon, tuna, and mackerel into your diet can be a game-changer. These fish are rich in omega-3s, which help reduce insulin resistance and support cardiovascular health, making them an essential part of a balanced, blood-sugar-friendly diet.

Grilled Salmon with Lemon and Asparagus

- Prep Time: 10 minutes
- Cook Time: 15 minutes
- Total Time: 25 minutes
- Servings: 2

INGREDIENTS :

- 2 salmon fillets (4 oz each)
- 1 tbsp olive oil
- 1 lemon, sliced
- 1 bunch asparagus, trimmed
- Salt and pepper, to taste
- 1 tsp fresh dill (optional)

NUTRITIONAL BREAKDOWN (PER SERVING):

- Calories: 380
- Carbs: 10g (3% of daily value)
- Protein: 35g (70% of daily value)
- Fiber: 5g (20% of daily value)
- Fats: 25g (38% of daily value)

HOW TO MAKE :

1. Preheat your grill or grill pan to medium heat.
2. Rub the salmon fillets with olive oil and season with salt and pepper.
3. Place the lemon slices on the grill and grill the salmon for 4-5 minutes per side, or until cooked through and the internal temperature reaches 145°F (63°C).
4. While the salmon is grilling, toss the asparagus with olive oil, salt, and pepper, and grill for 5-7 minutes, or until tender.
5. Serve the grilled salmon alongside the asparagus, garnished with fresh dill and a squeeze of grilled lemon.

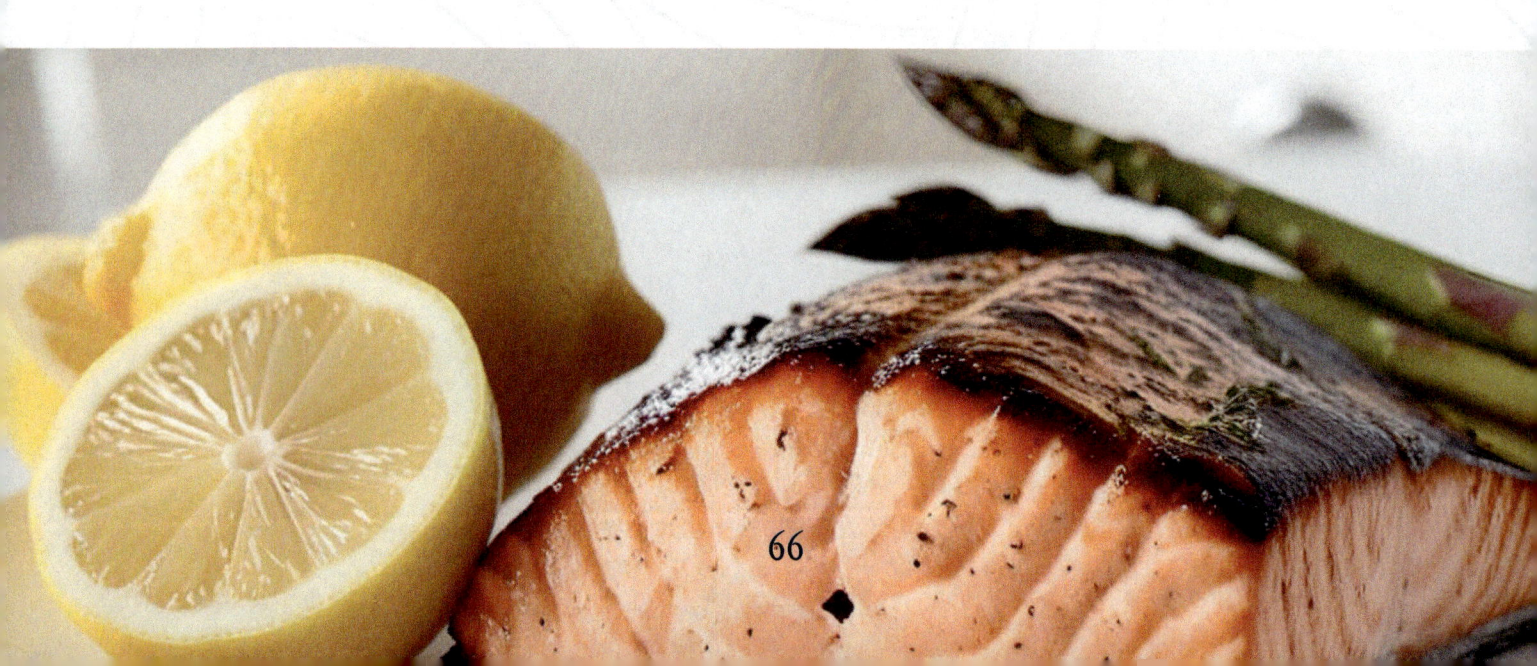

Baked Cod with Lemon-Caper Sauce

- Prep Time: 5 minutes
- Cook Time: 20 minutes
- Total Time: 25 minutes
- Servings: 2

INGREDIENTS :

- 2 cod fillets (4 oz each)
- 1 tbsp olive oil
- 1 lemon, juiced
- 1 tbsp capers, drained
- 1/4 cup fresh parsley, chopped
- Salt and pepper, to taste

NUTRITIONAL BREAKDOWN (PER SERVING):

- Calories: 220
- Carbs: 6g (2% of daily value)
- Protein: 30g (60% of daily value)
- Fiber: 2g (8% of daily value)
- Fats: 9g (14% of daily value)

HOW TO MAKE :

1. Preheat the oven to 375°F (190°C). Place the cod fillets on a baking sheet lined with parchment paper.
2. Drizzle the fillets with olive oil and season with salt and pepper.
3. Bake for 15-20 minutes, or until the cod flakes easily with a fork.
4. While the cod is baking, combine the lemon juice, capers, and fresh parsley in a small bowl.
5. Once the cod is cooked, pour the lemon-caper sauce over the fillets and serve immediately.

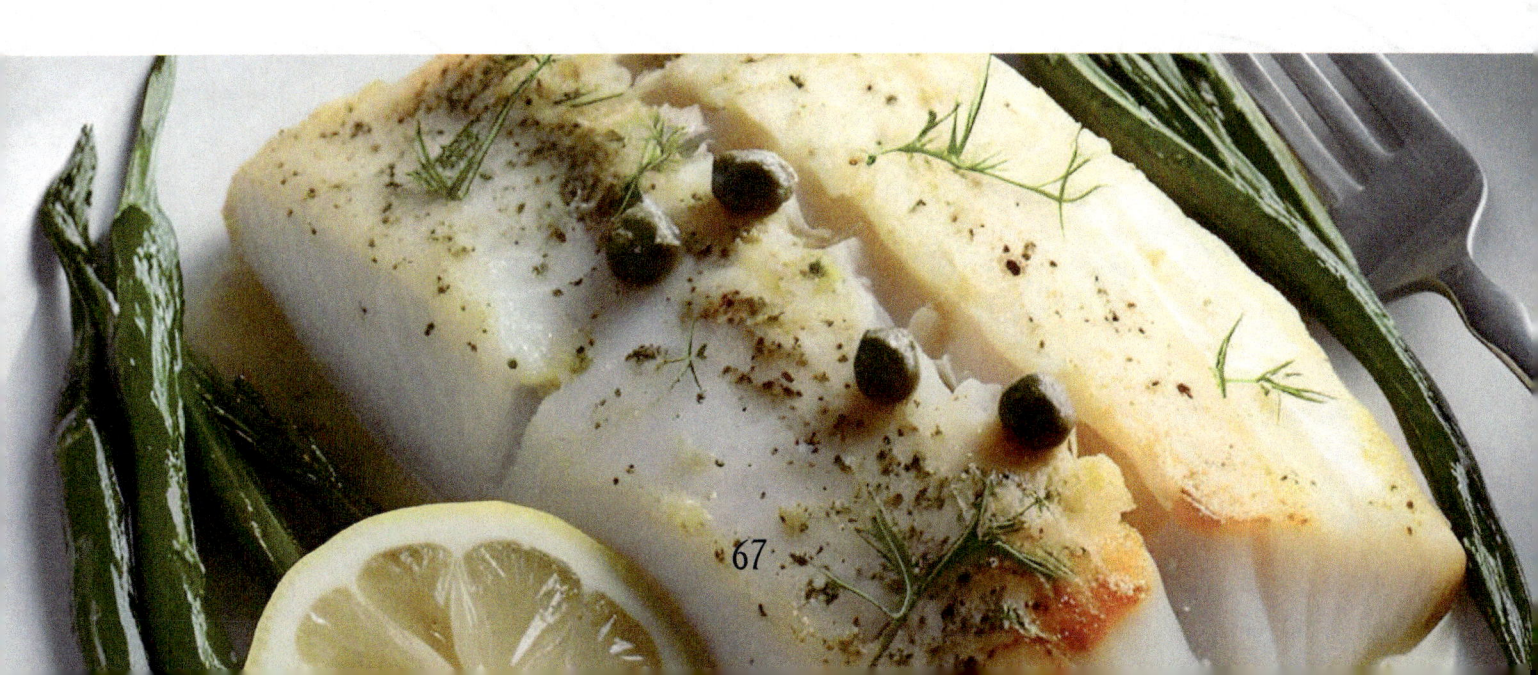

Shrimp and Avocado Salad with Cilantro-Lime Dressing

- Prep Time: 10 minutes
- Cook Time: 5 minutes
- Total Time: 15 minutes
- Servings: 2

INGREDIENTS :

- 1/2 lb shrimp, peeled and deveined
- 1 tbsp olive oil
- 1 avocado, diced
- 1/2 cup cherry tomatoes, halved
- 1/4 cup red onion, finely chopped
- 2 cups mixed greens (arugula, spinach, or lettuce)

FOR THE CILANTRO-LIME DRESSING:

- 2 tbsp fresh cilantro, chopped
- 1 tbsp lime juice
- 1 tbsp olive oil
- 1/2 tsp honey or stevia
- Salt and pepper, to taste

HOW TO MAKE :

1. Heat olive oil in a pan over medium-high heat. Add the shrimp and cook for 2-3 minutes per side, until pink and opaque. Remove from heat.
2. In a large bowl, combine the mixed greens, diced avocado, cherry tomatoes, and red onion.
3. For the dressing, whisk together cilantro, lime juice, olive oil, honey, salt, and pepper.
4. Add the cooked shrimp to the salad, drizzle with the cilantro-lime dressing, and toss gently to combine.
5. Serve immediately for a refreshing, protein-packed salad.

NUTRITIONAL BREAKDOWN (PER SERVING):

- Calories: 320
- Carbs: 14g (5% of daily value)
- Protein: 25g (50% of daily value)
- Fiber: 8g (32% of daily value)
- Fats: 22g (34% of daily value)

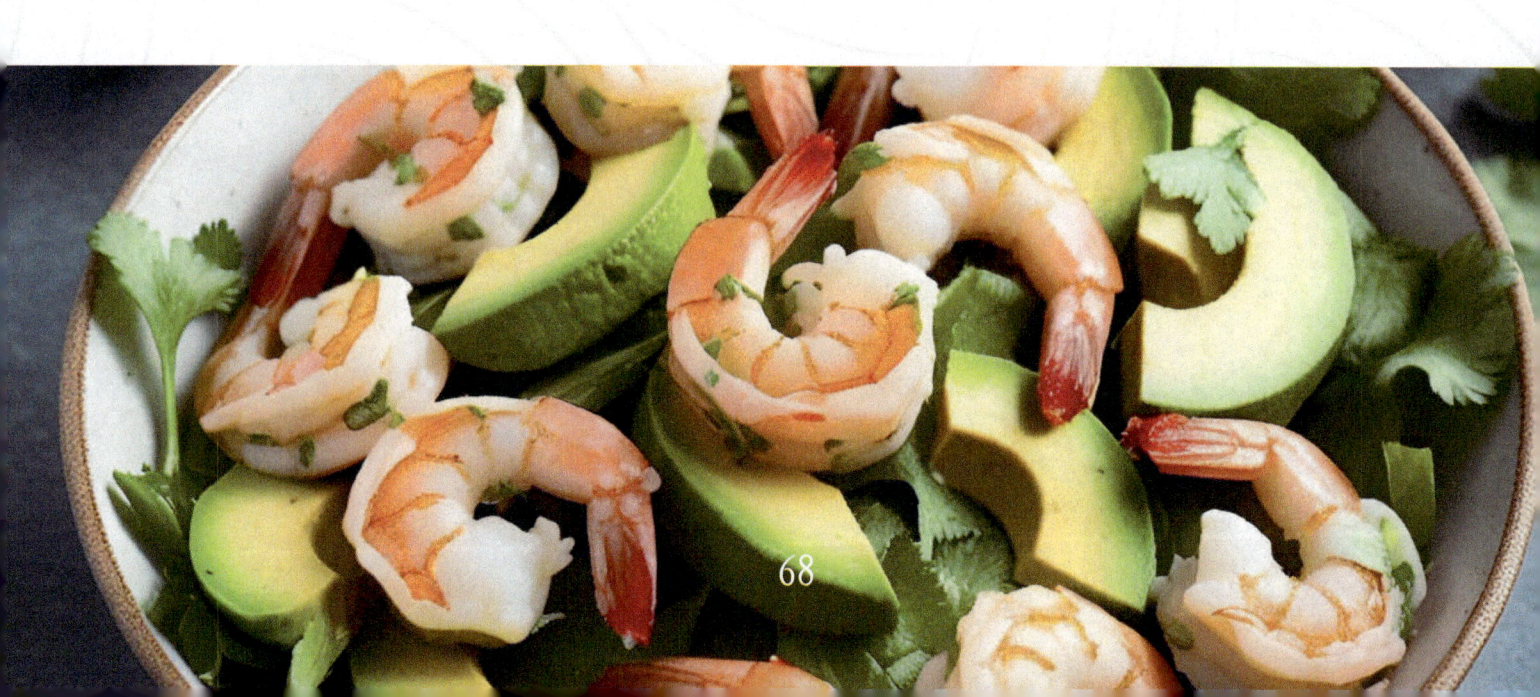

Lemon Herb Tilapia with Roasted Vegetables

- Prep Time: 10 minutes
- Cook Time: 20 minutes
- Total Time: 30 minutes
- Servings: 2

INGREDIENTS :

- 2 tilapia fillets (4 oz each)
- 1 tbsp olive oil
- 1 lemon, sliced
- 1 tsp dried oregano
- 1/2 tsp garlic powder
- Salt and pepper, to taste
- 1 cup Brussels sprouts, halved
- 1 medium sweet potato, cubed
- 1 tbsp olive oil (for roasting)
- Fresh parsley, for garnish

NUTRITIONAL BREAKDOWN (PER SERVING):

- Calories: 380
- Carbs: 35g (12% of daily value)
- Protein: 32g (64% of daily value)
- Fiber: 10g (40% of daily value)
- Fats: 16g (24% of daily value)

HOW TO MAKE :

1. Preheat the oven to 400°F (200°C). Place the tilapia fillets on a baking sheet lined with parchment paper.
2. Drizzle the tilapia with olive oil and sprinkle with oregano, garlic powder, salt, and pepper. Lay lemon slices on top of each fillet.
3. Toss the Brussels sprouts and sweet potato cubes with olive oil, salt, and pepper, and arrange them around the fish on the baking sheet.
4. Roast for 18-20 minutes, or until the tilapia flakes easily with a fork and the vegetables are tender.
5. Garnish with fresh parsley and serve warm.

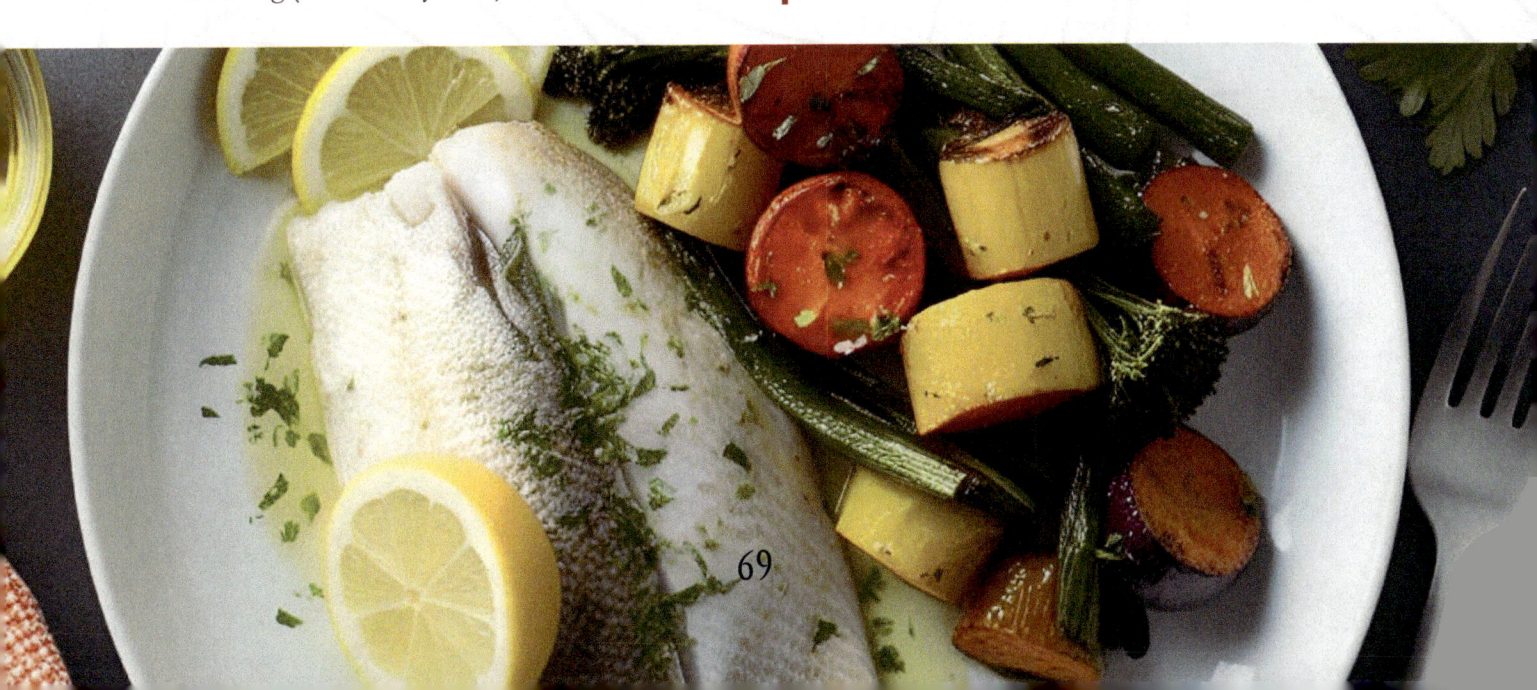

Tuna Salad Lettuce Wraps

- Prep Time: 10 minutes
- Cook Time: None
- Total Time: 10 minutes
- Servings: 2

INGREDIENTS :

- 1 can (5 oz) tuna in water, drained
- 1/4 cup plain Greek yogurt (unsweetened)
- 1 tbsp Dijon mustard
- 1 tbsp lemon juice
- 1/4 cup celery, diced
- 1/4 cup red onion, finely chopped
- Salt and pepper, to taste
- 6 large lettuce leaves (Romaine or Butter lettuce)

NUTRITIONAL BREAKDOWN (PER SERVING):

- Calories: 250
- Carbs: 6g (2% of daily value)
- Protein: 30g (60% of daily value)
- Fiber: 2g (8% of daily value)
- Fats: 12g (18% of daily value)

HOW TO MAKE :

1. In a bowl, combine the tuna, Greek yogurt, Dijon mustard, lemon juice, diced celery, red onion, salt, and pepper. Stir until well mixed.
2. Spoon the tuna salad into each lettuce leaf, creating a low-carb, crunchy wrap.
3. Serve immediately as a light and refreshing snack or meal.

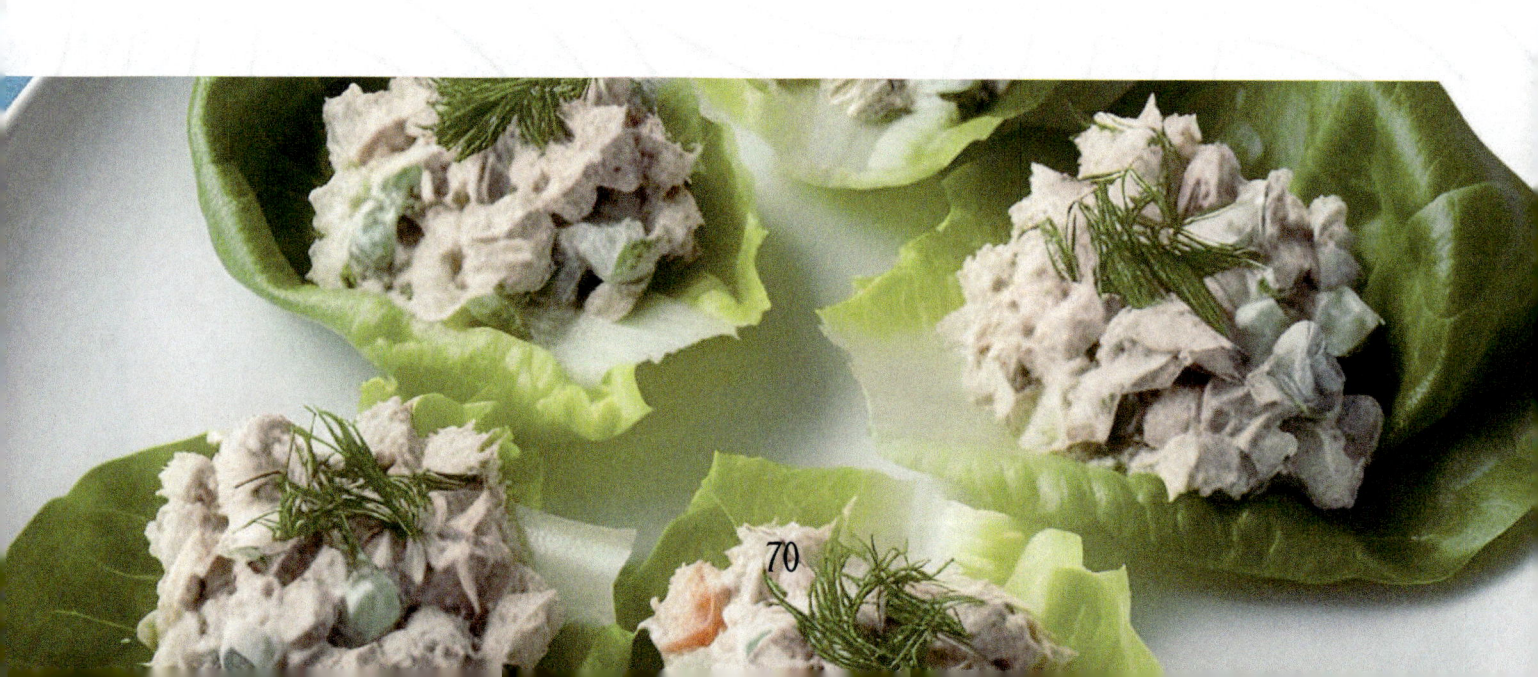

Grilled Mahi-Mahi with Mango Salsa

- Prep Time: 10 minutes
- Cook Time: 15 minutes
- Total Time: 25 minutes
- Servings: 2

INGREDIENTS :

- 2 mahi-mahi fillets (4 oz each)
- 1 tbsp olive oil
- Salt and pepper, to taste
- 1 ripe mango, diced
- 1/4 cup red onion, diced
- 1/4 cup cilantro, chopped
- 1 tbsp lime juice
- 1/4 tsp chili flakes (optional)

NUTRITIONAL BREAKDOWN (PER SERVING):

- Calories: 320
- Carbs: 20g (7% of daily value)
- Protein: 30g (60% of daily value)
- Fiber: 6g (24% of daily value)
- Fats: 16g (24% of daily value)

HOW TO MAKE :

1. Preheat the grill or grill pan to medium heat. Drizzle the mahi-mahi fillets with olive oil and season with salt and pepper.
2. Grill the fillets for about 4-5 minutes per side, or until the fish is opaque and flakes easily with a fork.
3. While the fish is grilling, prepare the mango salsa: In a bowl, combine the diced mango, red onion, cilantro, lime juice, and chili flakes (if using).
4. Serve the grilled mahi-mahi topped with the fresh mango salsa for a zesty and refreshing dish.

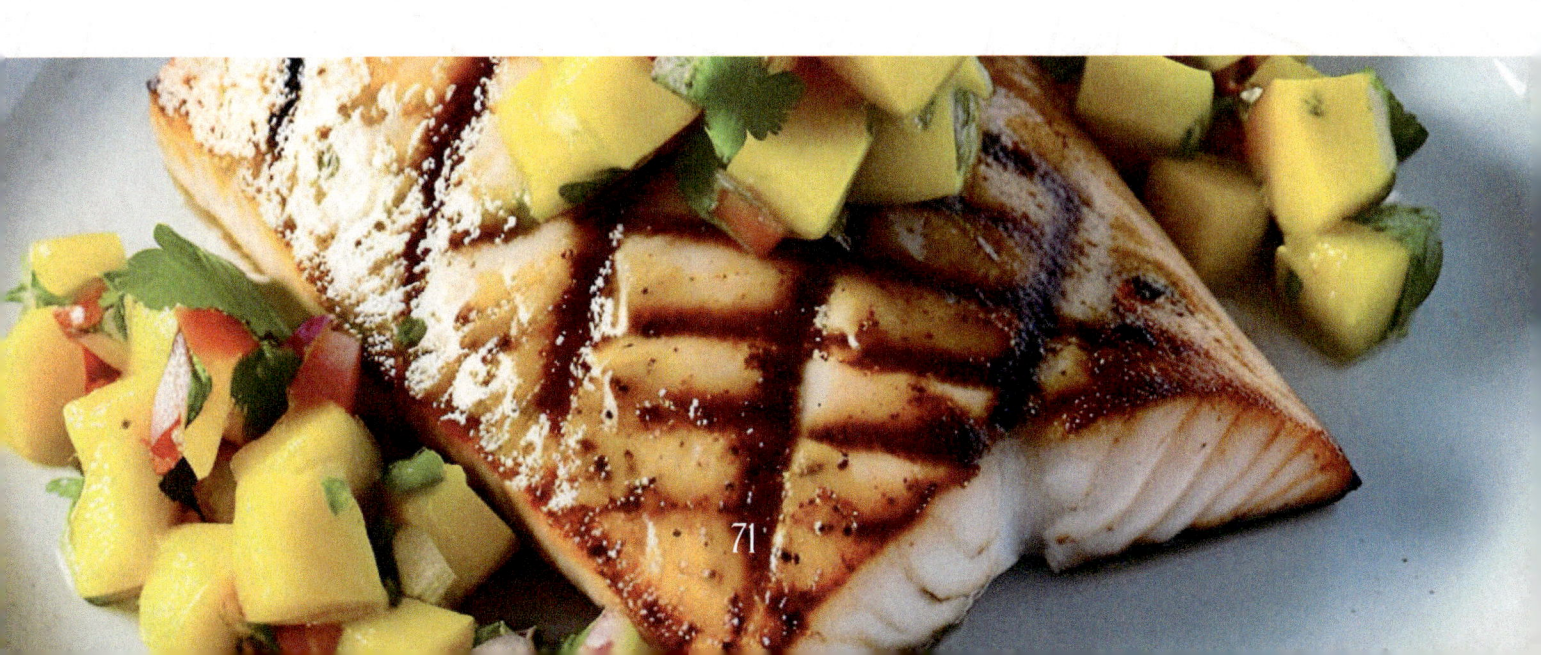

Shrimp Stir-Fry with Bell Peppers and Quinoa

- Prep Time: 10 minutes
- Cook Time: 15 minutes
- Total Time: 25 minutes
- Servings: 2

INGREDIENTS :

- 1/2 lb shrimp, peeled and deveined
- 1 tbsp olive oil
- 1 red bell pepper, sliced
- 1/2 cup zucchini, sliced
- 1/4 cup onion, sliced
- 1 cup cooked quinoa
- 2 tbsp low-sodium soy sauce
- 1 tsp sesame oil
- 1/2 tsp garlic powder
- 1 tbsp fresh cilantro, chopped (optional)

NUTRITIONAL BREAKDOWN (PER SERVING):

- Calories: 350
- Carbs: 35g (12% of daily value)
- Protein: 30g (60% of daily value)
- Fiber: 6g (24% of daily value)
- Fats: 15g (23% of daily value)

HOW TO MAKE :

1. Heat olive oil in a skillet over medium-high heat. Add the shrimp and cook for 2-3 minutes per side, until pink and opaque. Remove from the skillet and set aside.
2. In the same skillet, add the bell pepper, zucchini, and onion. Stir-fry for 3-5 minutes, until the vegetables are tender-crisp.
3. Add the cooked quinoa, soy sauce, sesame oil, and garlic powder to the skillet. Stir to combine and cook for an additional 2-3 minutes to warm through.
4. Return the cooked shrimp to the skillet and toss everything together. Garnish with fresh cilantro, if desired, and serve immediately.

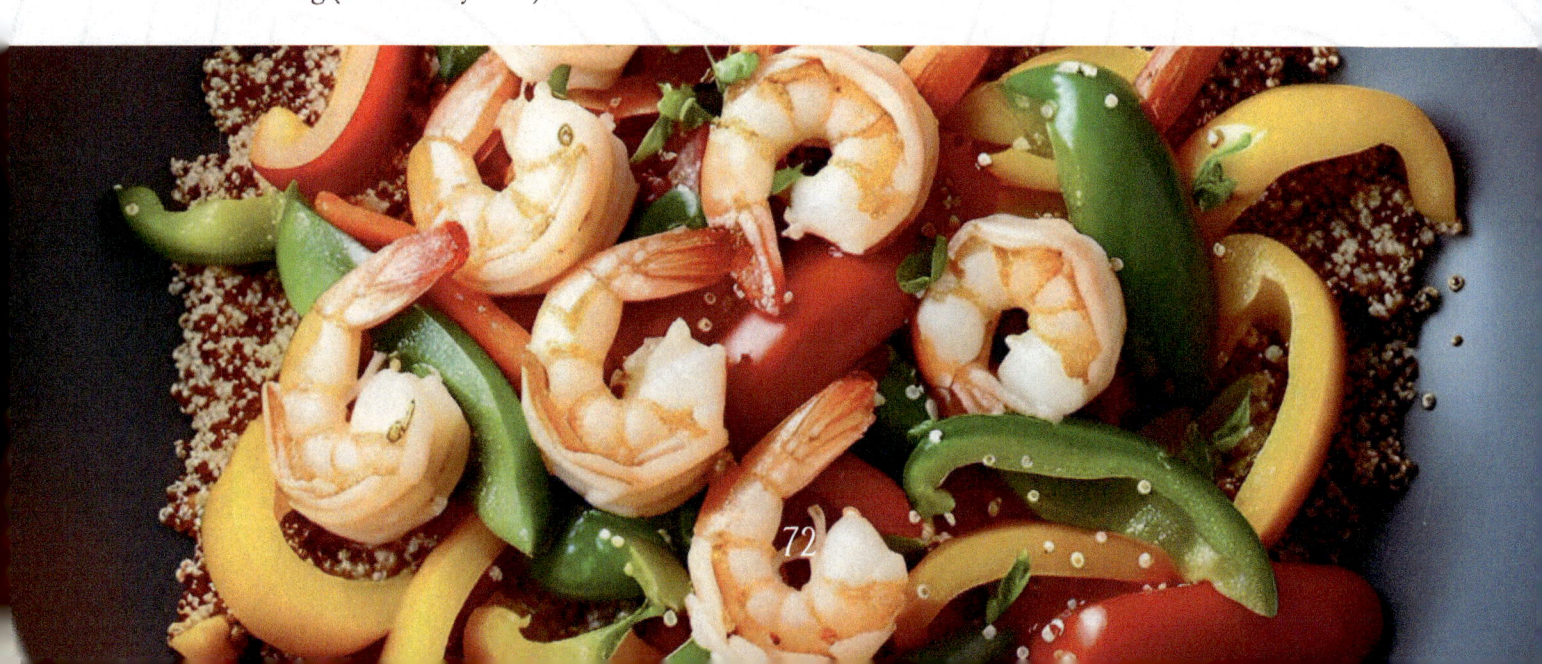

Baked Sea Bass with Olive Oil and Fresh Herbs

- Prep Time: 10 minutes
- Cook Time: 20 minutes
- Total Time: 30 minutes
- Servings: 2

INGREDIENTS :

- 2 sea bass fillets (4 oz each)
- 1 tbsp olive oil
- 1 tbsp lemon juice
- 1 tsp fresh thyme, chopped
- 1 tsp fresh rosemary, chopped
- Salt and pepper, to taste
- 1 lemon, sliced

NUTRITIONAL BREAKDOWN (PER SERVING):

- Calories: 280
- Carbs: 4g (1% of daily value)
- Protein: 35g (70% of daily value)
- Fiber: 2g (8% of daily value)
- Fats: 14g (22% of daily value)

HOW TO MAKE :

1. Preheat the oven to 375°F (190°C). Place the sea bass fillets on a baking sheet lined with parchment paper.
2. Drizzle the fillets with olive oil and lemon juice. Sprinkle with fresh thyme, rosemary, salt, and pepper.
3. Lay the lemon slices over the top of the fillets.
4. Bake for 15-20 minutes, or until the fish flakes easily with a fork.
5. Serve warm with extra lemon wedges on the side.

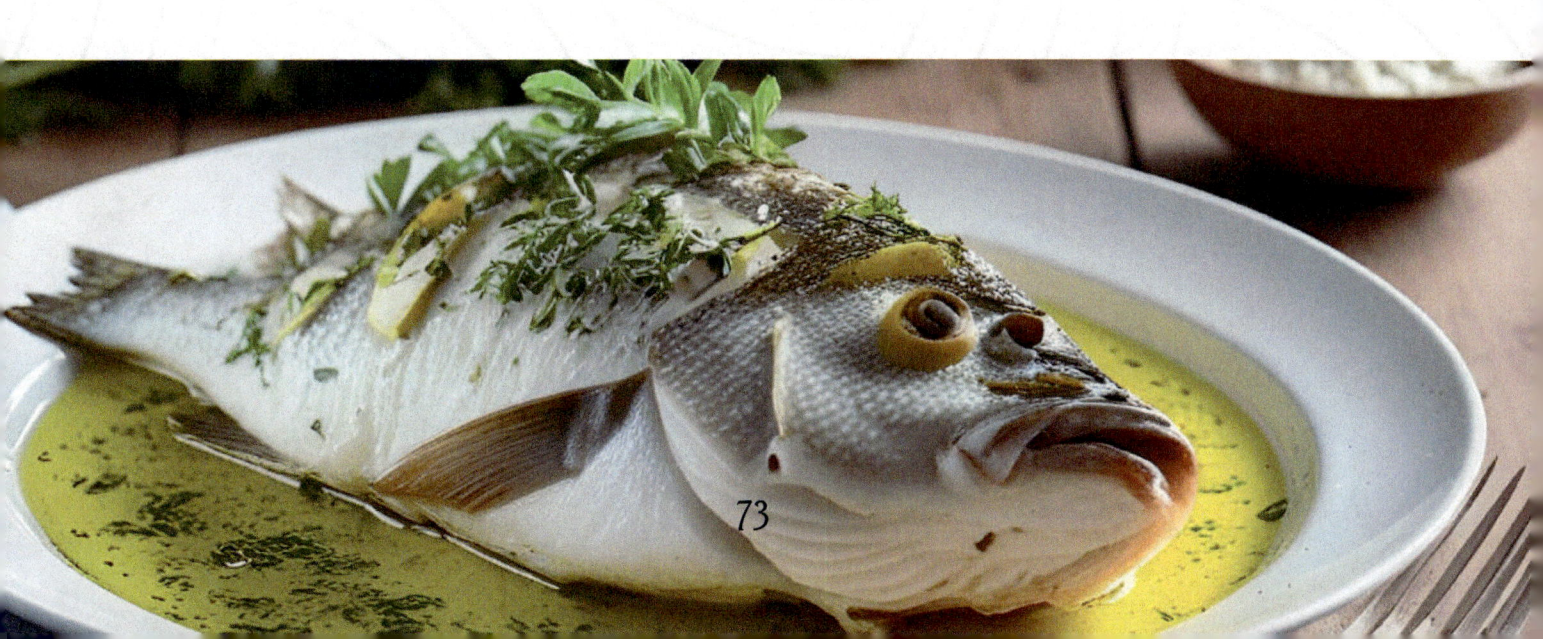

Chapter 9: What to Eat for Prediabetes Management

Managing prediabetes doesn't have to feel overwhelming, especially when you embrace a diet filled with whole foods that support stable blood sugar and overall health. This chapter will focus on the best foods to include in your diet, which will not only help manage blood sugar but also promote long-term wellness. The foods discussed here are packed with fiber, healthy fats, lean proteins, and antioxidants all essential for managing prediabetes effectively.

Whether you're just starting your journey to better health or you're looking to fine-tune your diet, these simple yet powerful foods will help you feel energized and in control. Let's explore the foods that should be at the top of your grocery list.

THE BEST FOODS TO INCLUDE IN YOUR DIET

Non-Starchy Vegetables
Non-starchy vegetables are your go-to foods when it comes to controlling blood sugar. They are naturally low in carbs and high in fiber, both of which help slow the digestion of carbohydrates and prevent blood sugar spikes.

Examples:
- Leafy greens (spinach, kale, arugula)
- Broccoli and cauliflower
- Zucchini and cucumbers
- Bell peppers and tomatoes
- Asparagus and green beans

Why they work for prediabetes:
These vegetables are nutrient-dense and full of antioxidants, which help reduce inflammation and promote overall health. The fiber in non-starchy vegetables slows sugar absorption and keeps blood sugar levels steady throughout the day.

Shopping Tip:
Stock up on fresh or frozen non-starchy vegetables to keep your meals easy to prepare. Try buying in bulk when possible to save money, and experiment with different herbs and spices to add flavor.

WHOLE GRAINS AND FIBER-RICH FOODS

Whole grains are packed with fiber, which is crucial for managing blood sugar levels. Unlike refined grains, whole grains provide a steady release of energy, preventing rapid spikes and crashes in blood sugar.

Examples:
- Quinoa
- Brown rice
- Oats (steel-cut or rolled)
- Barley
- Whole-wheat pasta
- Farro

Why they work for prediabetes:
Whole grains are rich in fiber, which helps improve insulin sensitivity and keeps blood sugar levels more consistent. They also provide essential B vitamins and minerals that support your metabolism and energy levels.

Shopping Tip:
Look for whole-grain products that list "whole wheat" or "whole grain" as the first ingredient. Opt for brown rice over white rice and oats without added sugars. Experiment with different grains like quinoa and farro for variety in your meals.

LEAN PROTEINS

Proteins are essential for building and repairing tissues, and lean protein sources help stabilize blood sugar without adding unhealthy fats.

Examples:
- Chicken breast (skinless)
- Turkey (ground or breast)
- Fish (salmon, mackerel, cod)
- Eggs
- Tofu and tempeh
- Legumes (lentils, chickpeas, black beans)

Why they work for prediabetes:
Lean proteins help keep you feeling full and satisfied, preventing overeating and reducing blood sugar spikes after meals. The omega-3 fatty acids found in fatty fish like salmon also improve insulin sensitivity and reduce inflammation.

Shopping Tip:
Choose skinless poultry and fish for lower fat content. Look for canned beans with no added salt and stock up on frozen fish for convenience.

HEALTHY FATS

Contrary to popular belief, healthy fats are essential for managing blood sugar and supporting heart health. These fats help reduce inflammation and improve insulin sensitivity.

Examples:
- Avocados
- Olive oil and canola oil
- Nuts (almonds, walnuts, pistachios)
- Seeds (chia, flax, pumpkin)
- Fatty fish (salmon, sardines, mackerel)

Why they work for prediabetes:
Healthy fats help you feel full and support blood sugar balance. They also improve cholesterol levels and reduce inflammation, all of which are crucial for long-term health.

Shopping Tip:
Keep avocados and nuts on hand for easy, nutrient-dense snacks. Olive oil should be your go-to cooking oil, and make sure to include fatty fish in your weekly meals for the benefits of omega-3 fatty acids.

LOW-GLYCEMIC FRUITS

Fruits are an important part of a healthy diet, but low-glycemic fruits have the added benefit of causing a slower, more gradual rise in blood sugar levels. These fruits are full of fiber, vitamins, and antioxidants.

Examples:
- Berries (strawberries, blueberries, raspberries)
- Apples
- Pears
- Peaches
- Cherries

Why they work for prediabetes:
Low-glycemic fruits provide vitamins, fiber, and antioxidants without causing rapid blood sugar spikes. They are also a great source of polyphenols, which have been shown to improve insulin sensitivity.

Shopping Tip:
Choose fresh or frozen berries for a low-sugar option. Apples and pears are easy-to-carry snacks that keep you feeling full longer due to their high fiber content.

SUPERFOODS FOR PREDIABETES

Certain superfoods are especially beneficial for blood sugar regulation. These foods contain high levels of antioxidants, anti-inflammatory properties, and nutrients that help improve insulin sensitivity and reduce inflammation.

CINNAMON, TURMERIC, AND GINGER

These spices have been shown to improve insulin sensitivity and reduce inflammation in the body.
- **Cinnamon:** May help lower blood sugar and improve insulin sensitivity.
- **Turmeric:** Contains curcumin, which has powerful anti-inflammatory effects and may help improve insulin resistance.
- **Ginger:** Known for its anti-inflammatory properties and may help lower blood sugar levels.

How to use:
- Sprinkle cinnamon on your oatmeal, smoothies, or baked goods. Add turmeric to soups, stews, or rice dishes. Use fresh ginger in smoothies, stir-fries, or hot tea.

BERRIES, NUTS, AND SEEDS

These foods are rich in antioxidants, fiber, and healthy fats that support blood sugar control and heart health.

- **Berries:** Packed with fiber and antioxidants, berries are perfect for snacking or adding to smoothies and salads.
- **Nuts:** Almonds, walnuts, and pistachios are great sources of healthy fats and protein, which help regulate blood sugar.
- **Seeds:** Chia seeds, flaxseeds, and pumpkin seeds are rich in fiber and omega-3s, which support blood sugar regulation and satiety.

How to use:
Add berries to your yogurt or oatmeal. Enjoy a handful of nuts as a snack. Use seeds in salads, smoothies, or as a topping for your favorite dishes.

LEAFY GREENS

Leafy greens like spinach, kale, and arugula are low in carbs and high in fiber, vitamins, and minerals. These greens help manage blood sugar and promote overall digestive health.

- **Spinach:** Rich in vitamins A, C, and K, and folate.
- **Kale:** Packed with fiber, antioxidants, and calcium.
- **Arugula:** A peppery green full of vitamin C and fiber.

<u>How to use:</u>
- Add leafy greens to salads, sandwiches, soups, or smoothies for a nutrient-dense boost.

EASY-TO-MAKE, PREDIABETES-FRIENDLY SNACKS

Healthy snacks are key to maintaining balanced blood sugar levels throughout the day. Here are some simple, blood-sugar-friendly snack ideas:

- Apple slices with almond butter
- Carrot sticks with hummus
- Greek yogurt with chia seeds and berries
- Hard-boiled eggs with a sprinkle of paprika
- A handful of mixed nuts

As you shop for these foods, remember to buy in bulk where possible and stick to fresh, whole foods that are free from added sugars and preservatives. The goal is to make these healthy foods a regular part of your diet, creating a sustainable, enjoyable, and blood-sugar-friendly lifestyle.

By embracing these foods, you'll be on your way to feeling your best and managing prediabetes with ease, all while enjoying flavorful, satisfying meals. Happy eating!

Bonus: Your 28-Day Meal Plan (Jumpstart Your Journey to Better Health)

Starting your journey toward better blood sugar management can feel overwhelming at first, but with the right plan in place, it becomes not only achievable but also enjoyable. This 28-day meal plan is designed to help you take control of your health by incorporating balanced meals that are nutrient-dense, delicious, and blood-sugar friendly.

Each meal plan is designed to nourish and energize, so you can take the first steps towards healthier living with confidence and support. Let's dive into how this meal plan works and how you can make it a sustainable part of your routine.

Week 1: Reset and Refuel

DAY	BREAKFAST	LUNCH	DINNER	SNACK
DAY 1	SCRAMBLED EGGS WITH SPINACH AND AVOCADO	GRILLED CHICKEN WITH QUINOA AND BROCCOLI	SALMON WITH ROASTED ASPARAGUS AND SWEET POTATO	GREEK YOGURT WITH CHIA SEEDS
DAY 2	OATMEAL WITH CHIA SEEDS AND BERRIES	QUINOA SALAD WITH CUCUMBER, TOMATO, AND MINT	GRILLED TURKEY WITH ROASTED BRUSSELS SPROUTS	A HANDFUL OF ALMONDS
DAY 3	GREEN SMOOTHIE WITH SPINACH, BANANA, AND FLAXSEEDS	LENTIL SOUP WITH KALE AND CARROTS	BAKED COD WITH A SIDE OF ROASTED CAULIFLOWER	CELERY STICKS WITH HUMMUS
DAY 4	AVOCADO TOAST WITH POACHED EGG ON WHOLE GRAIN BREAD	CHICKEN AND VEGETABLE STIR-FRY WITH BROWN RICE	SHRIMP AND VEGETABLE SKEWERS WITH QUINOA	APPLE SLICES WITH ALMOND BUTTER
DAY 5	CHIA PUDDING WITH BERRIES	TURKEY LETTUCE WRAPS WITH AVOCADO	GRILLED TILAPIA WITH ZUCCHINI AND ROASTED CARROTS	HARD-BOILED EGGS
DAY 6	GREEK YOGURT WITH MIXED BERRIES	VEGGIE-PACKED SALAD WITH GRILLED CHICKEN	BAKED CHICKEN WITH MASHED CAULIFLOWER AND SPINACH	CARROT STICKS WITH GUACAMOLE
DAY 7	COTTAGE CHEESE WITH CUCUMBER AND TOMATOES	TUNA SALAD WITH LEAFY GREENS AND OLIVE OIL DRESSING	GRILLED SALMON WITH STEAMED BROCCOLI	A HANDFUL OF MIXED NUTS

Week 2: Building Healthy Habits

DAY	BREAKFAST	LUNCH	DINNER	SNACK
DAY 8	SCRAMBLED TOFU WITH VEGGIES AND WHOLE GRAIN TOAST	GRILLED CHICKEN WITH QUINOA AND ROASTED VEGETABLES	BAKED SALMON WITH SWEET POTATO AND STEAMED ASPARAGUS	A HANDFUL OF WALNUTS
DAY 9	GREEK YOGURT WITH CHIA SEEDS AND STRAWBERRIES	LENTIL AND VEGETABLE STEW WITH A SIDE OF BROWN RICE	GRILLED CHICKEN WITH A SIDE OF ROASTED BRUSSELS SPROUTS	CARROT AND CELERY STICKS WITH HUMMUS
DAY 10	SMOOTHIE WITH SPINACH, ALMOND MILK, BANANA, AND PROTEIN POWDER	SPINACH AND STRAWBERRY SALAD WITH WALNUTS	SPAGHETTI SQUASH WITH PESTO AND CHERRY TOMATOES	A HARD-BOILED EGG
DAY 11	OATMEAL WITH ALMOND BUTTER AND SLICED BANANAS	CHICKPEA SALAD WITH AVOCADO AND A LEMON DRESSING	GRILLED SHRIMP WITH QUINOA AND GRILLED VEGETABLES	APPLE SLICES WITH ALMOND BUTTER
DAY 12	EGG AND VEGGIE SCRAMBLE WITH AVOCADO SLICES	GRILLED TURKEY WITH ROASTED SWEET POTATOES	TUNA SALAD WITH LEAFY GREENS AND OLIVE OIL DRESSING	GREEK YOGURT WITH BERRIES
DAY 13	WHOLE GRAIN TOAST WITH AVOCADO AND POACHED EGGS	QUINOA AND ROASTED VEGETABLE SALAD WITH LEMON-TAHINI DRESSING	BAKED COD WITH STEAMED BROCCOLI AND MASHED CAULIFLOWER	A HANDFUL OF ALMONDS
DAY 14	SMOOTHIE BOWL WITH BERRIES, ALMOND MILK, AND CHIA SEEDS	GRILLED CHICKEN AND AVOCADO SALAD WITH A LIME DRESSING	BAKED CHICKEN WITH ROASTED CARROTS AND SPINACH	VEGGIE STICKS WITH HUMMUS

Week 3: Sustaining Progress

DAY	BREAKFAST	LUNCH	DINNER	SNACK
DAY 15	SCRAMBLED EGGS WITH TOMATOES AND SPINACH	CHICKEN AND VEGGIE STIR-FRY WITH BROWN RICE	GRILLED SALMON WITH ROASTED BUTTERNUT SQUASH AND GREENS	HANDFUL OF ALMONDS AND A SMALL APPLE
DAY 16	CHIA PUDDING WITH MIXED BERRIES	LENTIL AND QUINOA SALAD WITH LEMON DRESSING	BAKED CHICKEN WITH ROASTED CAULIFLOWER AND BRUSSELS SPROUTS	CARROT STICKS WITH HUMMUS
DAY 17	VEGGIE-PACKED OMELETTE WITH AVOCADO	TUNA SALAD WITH LEAFY GREENS AND OLIVE OIL DRESSING	TURKEY MEATBALLS WITH SPAGHETTI SQUASH AND MARINARA SAUCE	GREEK YOGURT WITH CHIA SEEDS
DAY 18	SMOOTHIE WITH SPINACH, ALMOND MILK, AND CHIA SEEDS	GRILLED CHICKEN AND ROASTED SWEET POTATO SALAD	SHRIMP STIR-FRY WITH BELL PEPPERS AND QUINOA	CELERY WITH ALMOND BUTTER
DAY 19	AVOCADO TOAST WITH POACHED EGGS	QUINOA AND CHICKPEA SALAD WITH CUCUMBER AND MINT	BAKED COD WITH LEMON AND ROASTED VEGETABLES	A HANDFUL OF MIXED NUTS
DAY 20	OATMEAL WITH GROUND FLAXSEED AND BERRIES	TURKEY LETTUCE WRAPS WITH AVOCADO AND TOMATO	CAULIFLOWER RICE STIR-FRY WITH TOFU AND VEGETABLES	SLICED CUCUMBER WITH GUACAMOLE
DAY 21	GREEK YOGURT WITH WALNUTS AND BERRIES	SPINACH AND STRAWBERRY SALAD WITH BALSAMIC DRESSING	BAKED SALMON WITH A SIDE OF STEAMED ASPARAGUS	HARD-BOILED EGG AND CARROT STICKS

Week 4: Mastering Your Blood Sugar

DAY	BREAKFAST	LUNCH	DINNER	SNACK
DAY 22	Green smoothie with avocado and chia seed	Roasted chicken and quinoa salad with cucumbers and feta	Grilled tilapia with roasted sweet potatoes and broccoli	Apple slices with peanut butter
DAY 23	Oats with almond butter and mixed berries	Grilled turkey burger with avocado on a lettuce bun	Shrimp scampi with zucchini noodles	A handful of pumpkin seeds
DAY 24	Scrambled eggs with sautéed mushrooms and spinach	Chickpea and spinach stew	Baked chicken with cauliflower mash and roasted carrots	Greek yogurt with flax seeds
DAY 25	Avocado toast with an egg	Spinach and feta salad with lemon dressing	Lemon garlic salmon with steamed green beans	Carrot sticks with guacamole
DAY 26	Chia pudding with blueberries and walnuts	Lentil soup with kale and quinoa	Turkey meatballs with roasted Brussels sprouts	A handful of mixed nuts
DAY 27	Smoothie with spinach, protein powder, and almond milk	Grilled chicken with roasted sweet potato	Grilled shrimp with vegetable stir-fry and quinoa	Celery with almond butter
DAY 28	Scrambled eggs with avocado and salsa	Quinoa and roasted vegetable salad	Baked salmon with roasted asparagus and quinoa	Hard-boiled egg and cucumber slices

GROCERY LIST FOR WEEK 1:

- Eggs, Greek yogurt, chia seeds, flaxseeds
- Fresh spinach, kale, broccoli, Brussels sprouts, cauliflower, zucchini, carrots
- Chicken breast, turkey breast, tilapia, cod, salmon, shrimp
- Avocados, cucumbers, tomatoes, mixed berries, apples
- Olive oil, quinoa, oats, whole grain bread, almond butter, mixed nuts
- Hummus, guacamole, cottage cheese

GROCERY LIST FOR WEEK 2:

- Tofu, chicken breast, turkey breast, salmon, shrimp, cod
- Avocados, spinach, kale, tomatoes, strawberries, bananas, apples
- Whole grain bread, oats, quinoa, brown rice
- Greek yogurt, chia seeds, almond butter, hummus, mixed nuts
- Sweet potatoes, carrots, broccoli, Brussels sprouts, zucchini
- Lemon, tahini, olive oil, protein powder

GROCERY LIST FOR WEEK 3:

- Eggs, Greek yogurt, chia seeds, flaxseeds
- Chicken breast, turkey breast, salmon, cod, shrimp
- Fresh spinach, kale, tomatoes, cucumbers, strawberries, berries, sweet potatoes, Brussels sprouts, cauliflower, bell peppers
- Quinoa, whole grain bread, oats, chickpeas, lentils, spaghetti squash
- Olive oil, balsamic vinegar, hummus, mixed nuts, walnuts, avocado

GROCERY LIST FOR WEEK 4:

- Eggs, Greek yogurt, chia seeds, flaxseeds, protein powder
- Chicken breast, turkey breast, tilapia, shrimp
- Fresh spinach, kale, tomatoes, cucumbers, sweet potatoes, broccoli, cauliflower, carrots, zucchini, Brussels sprouts, bell peppers, green beans
- Quinoa, oats, chickpeas, lentils, whole grain bread, mixed berries, apples, avocado
- Olive oil, balsamic vinegar, hummus, mixed nuts, walnuts, almond butter, peanut butter

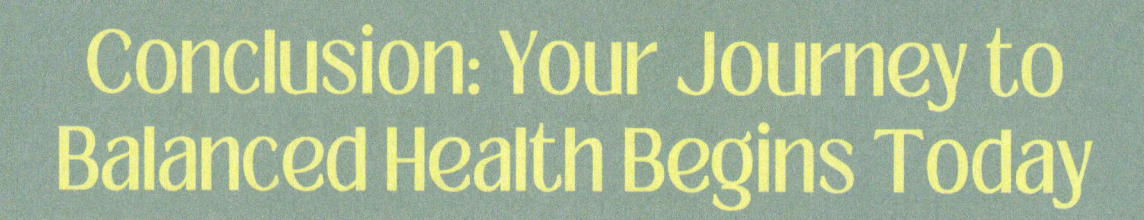

Conclusion: Your Journey to Balanced Health Begins Today

Thank you for joining me on this journey toward better health and blood sugar management. Whether you've been following this plan for a few days, weeks, or longer, you are already making positive changes in your life. Each step you've taken, no matter how small it may seem, is a victory in your journey to a healthier, more balanced lifestyle.

Managing prediabetes isn't about perfection it's about progress. It's about making small, consistent changes that, over time, add up to big results. You don't need to be perfect to succeed; you just need to stay committed to your health goals and take it one day at a time.

As you continue on this journey, remember that every meal, every healthy snack, and every small decision you make is a step in the right direction. By focusing on whole, nutrient-dense foods, staying active, and managing stress, you're giving yourself the best possible foundation for long-term wellness. You've already proven that you are capable of making lasting changes, and I have no doubt that you will continue to thrive.

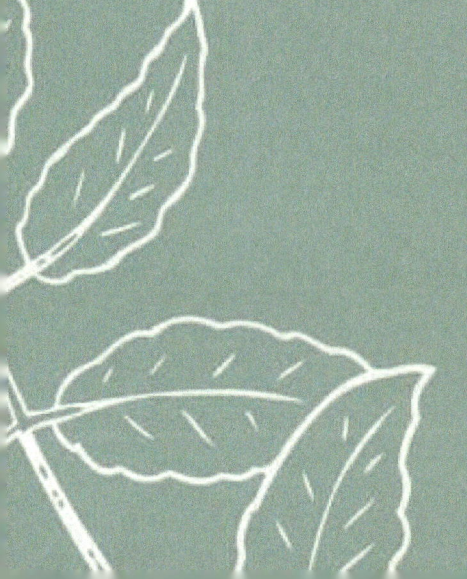

HOW TO CONTINUE ON YOUR PATH TO HEALTH AND WELLNESS

Now that you've completed the 28-day meal plan, the key is to keep building on what you've already accomplished. Consistency is the secret to continued success. Here's how to stay on track and make these healthy changes a permanent part of your lifestyle:

Celebrate Your Progress:
- Take a moment to reflect on how far you've come. Whether it's making better food choices, feeling more energized, or noticing positive changes in your health, celebrate those wins. Every step forward is a step toward your ultimate goal of balanced blood sugar and well-being.

Build on Your Healthy Habits:
- You've learned to embrace whole foods, manage portion sizes, and make healthier choices. Now, keep those habits going. Focus on variety in your meals, and don't be afraid to experiment with new recipes or foods that excite you. Remember, meal planning is a tool that helps make healthy eating easier. Use it as a guide but don't be afraid to adjust things as needed.

Incorporate Physical Activity:
- Exercise is a key component in managing prediabetes. Whether it's a brisk walk, yoga, or a workout routine you enjoy, staying active helps your body regulate blood sugar and improves overall health. Aim for at least 30 minutes of physical activity most days of the week and have fun with it! Find activities that make you feel good, and mix it up to keep it exciting.

Stay Hydrated and Mindful of Your Portions:
- It's easy to overlook the importance of staying hydrated, but drinking plenty of water throughout the day is essential for blood sugar regulation. Mind your portions and avoid overeating, even with healthy foods. Smaller, balanced meals throughout the day will help keep your blood sugar stable.

Connect with a Support System:
- Having a support system whether it's friends, family, or an online community can make all the difference. Surround yourself with people who are on a similar health journey, or who can offer encouragement when things get tough. You don't have to do this alone, and asking for help when needed is a sign of strength, not weakness.

REINFORCE THE MESSAGE: SMALL, CONSISTENT CHANGES LEAD TO BIG RESULTS

Managing prediabetes is a long-term commitment, but the small steps you've taken now are laying the groundwork for lasting success. These small, consistent changes will add up over time, creating big results. As you continue on your journey, focus on:

- Sustainability, not perfection
- Variety in your meals to keep things interesting.
- Consistency to stay committed to your health goals.

Remember, progress is not always linear, and there will be days when it feels like you've hit a plateau. But with patience, persistence, and the knowledge you've gained from this book, you'll find that these challenges are simply part of the process. You are building a foundation for long-term health and that's something to be incredibly proud of.

ENCOURAGE YOURSELF AND STAY COMMITTED TO YOUR HEALTH GOALS

You've already taken the most important step: deciding to take control of your health. Managing blood sugar, embracing a healthier lifestyle, and making better food choices is something to be proud of. As you continue on your path, remember to:

- Embrace progress over perfection this is a journey, not a race.
- Be patient with yourself and trust the process. The changes you're making will have lasting effects on your health.
- Stay committed to your goals, no matter how small they seem. Every positive change counts.

Thank you for allowing me to be part of your health journey. I'm proud of you for taking these steps, and I can't wait to see the continued progress you'll make. You've got this!Keep up the great work, and remember, this is just the beginning of your journey to better health! Keep experimenting with new recipes, stick with your healthy habits, and enjoy the benefits of a blood-sugar-friendly lifestyle!

Your health journey is just beginning, and with the tools, knowledge, and mindset you've developed, you are more than capable of achieving your wellness goals. Here's to the future of your health!

Printed in Dunstable, United Kingdom